2018—2019 年

中国老年医学学会
团体标准汇编

中国老年医学学会
国家老年疾病临床医学研究中心　编
（解放军总医院）

U0335668

中国标准出版社
北京

图书在版编目(CIP)数据

2018—2019年中国老年医学学会团体标准汇编/中国老年医学学会,国家老年疾病临床医学研究中心(解放军总医院)编. —北京:中国标准出版社,2020.9
ISBN 978-7-5066-9704-0

Ⅰ.①2… Ⅱ.①中…②国… Ⅲ.①老年病学—标准—汇编—中国 Ⅳ.①R592-65

中国版本图书馆 CIP 数据核字(2020)第 092200 号

中国标准出版社　出版发行
北京市朝阳区和平里西街甲 2 号(100029)
北京市西城区三里河北街 16 号(100045)
网址 www.spc.net.cn
总编室:(010)68533533　发行中心:(010)51780238
读者服务部:(010)68523946
中国标准出版社秦皇岛印刷厂印刷
各地新华书店经销

*

开本 880×1230 1/16　印张 12.25　字数 358 千字
2020 年 9 月第一版　2020 年 9 月第一次印刷

*

定价 180.00 元

前　言

　　截至 2018 年底,我国 60 岁以上人口达到 2.5 亿,占总人口的 17.9%,65 周岁及以上人口达到 1.7 亿,占总人口的 11.9%。我国人口老龄化达到较为严重的程度,已成为我国面临的一个极为严峻的社会问题。

　　习近平总书记在党的十九大报告中指出"实施健康中国战略,积极应对人口老龄化,构建养老、孝老、敬老政策体系和社会环境,推进医养结合,加快老龄事业和产业发展",为中国的老龄事业发展指明了方向。老龄事业前景光明,但是道路艰难。我国人口结构的老龄化是断崖式的发展轨迹,缺少政策体系化的应对措施,支撑老龄事业发展的标准基本处于空白状态。

　　中国老年医学学会(Chinese Geriatrics Society,CGS)于 2015 年 4 月 19 日在北京成立,是经中华人民共和国民政部(下简称民政部)注册批准的国家一级学会,是在民政部的领导、指导和监督管理下开展社会团体组织工作,是具有独立法人资格的全国性、行业性、公益性社会团体,是由从事老年医学预防、医疗、教学、科研、护理、康复、保健等专家、教授、学者自愿组成的学术组织。学会紧紧围绕国家全民健康战略和老年健康服务需求,按照"遵道敬医,健康生命"会训和"民主办会、科技强会、服务立会、开放兴会"理念,团结全体会员及全国老年医学和健康领域工作者积极响应国家政策,探索建立健康教育、预防保健、疾病诊治、技能培训、医养疗护服务体系,已形成覆盖全国的产学研用一体化老年健康服务新格局。

　　学会根据多年的调研总结认为,构建健康、医疗与照护相支撑,机构、社区与家庭相结合的医养服务体系是应对人口老龄化的有效举措。为此,中国老年医学学会本着"技术推动、标准先行,政府主导、行业共建,社会共治、全民共享"的发展目标,制定完善社会所需的相关适老标准,逐步构建适老标准体系。

　　什么是适老标准体系? 标准是通过标准化活动,按照规定的程序经协商一致制定,为各种活动或其结果提供规则、指南或特性,供共同使用和重复使用的文件。标准以科学、技术和实践经验的综合成果为基础,以促进最佳社会效益为目的,是经济活动和社会发展的技术支撑。一定范围内的标准按其内在联系形成的科学有机整体就是标准体系。适老标准体系就是围绕老年人衣食住行医的生活需求,科学制定的"适合老年人群"健康需求的标准体系。

　　为了科学、高效的制定出符合当前社会急需的适老相关标准,中国老年医学学会充分发挥学会在医学、养老、营养、康复、照护等方面的学术优势,成立了标准化管理部,聘请国家权威标准化专家参与制定本会团体标准的发展战略规划,指导和培训标准撰写者相关业务。学会在每项标准立项、起草和审查过程中都邀请有经验的专家、机构代表参与,组成专业能力强、覆盖范围广的专家团队,充分结合行业发展实际情况,广泛征求意见,力求制定科学实用的适老标准。

本书汇编了2018—2019年中国老年医学学会发布实施的6项适老相关团体标准,包括 T/CGSS 001—2018《老年照护师规范》、T/CGSS 003—2019《老年友善服务规范》、T/CGSS 004—2019《适老营养配方食品通则》、T/CGSS 005—2019《医养结合服务机构设施设置基本要求》、T/CGSS 006—2019《医养结合服务机构等级评定规范》和 T/CGSS 007—2019《社区适老营养师规范》。这6项标准都已在"全国团体标准信息平台"上发布。

6项标准互为依托、相互支撑,形成了健康医养的局部体系,可为相关企事业单位发展老龄化事业提供技术支持。关于团体标准的推广及应用,学会将在政府相关主管部门的指导下,与社会各界加强合作,共同构建科学合理的健康医养标准体系。就具体标准而言,学会邀请了国内知名企业参与达成了优先应用、共同推广的战略合作意向。

少年强则国家强,老年安则社会安。关心关爱老年群体,需要政府和全社会的共同努力,中国老年医学学会积极配合国家老年健康服务体系建设,主动引领健康老龄化科技发展,推进医养科学结合、适老科技成果转化、老年健康教育工作。愿竭诚为健康事业服务,维护老年健康和生命尊严,遵道敬医,恪尽职守,努力奉献!

编　者

2020 年 5 月

目　　录

ICS 03.080
A 20

团 体 标 准

T/CGSS 001—2018

老 年 照 护 师 规 范

Specification for elderly caregiver

2018-11-01 发布

2018-11-01 实施

中国老年医学学会　发 布

前　言

本标准按照 GB/T 1.1—2009 给出的规则起草。

本标准由中国老年医学学会老年医疗照护分会提出。

本标准由中国老年医学学会归口。

本标准起草单位:中国老年医学学会老年医疗照护分会、解放军总医院、北京协和医院、北京老年医院、浙江大学医学院附属第一医院、陆军军医大学、中国医科大学附属盛京医院、第二军医大学长海医院、湖南省肿瘤医院、南方医科大学珠江医院、四川大学华西医院、解放军兰州总医院、辽宁省金秋医院、解放军沈阳军区总医院、宁波大学医学院附属医院、成都市第八人民医院、深圳大学心理与社会学院、重庆医科大学附属第一医院青杠老年护养中心、北京市丰台区康助养护院。

本标准主要起草人:皮红英、侯惠如、郭娜、邓宝凤、杨燕妮、朱斌、张勤、范玲、张玲娟、谌永毅、刘雪琴、胡秀英、陆皓、孔琳姝、胡学军、盛芝仁、胡建利、关青、喻秀丽、于安安、王晓媛、杨晶、石海燕、孙静、来纯云、刘玉春。

老 年 照 护 师 规 范

1 范围

本标准规定了老年照护师的分级、通用要求、职业要求、技能要求和考核。

本标准适用于老年照护师的培训、等级评定与考核。

2 术语和定义

下列术语和定义适用于本文件。

2.1

老年照护 elderly care

为部分或全部功能障碍的老年人提供系列健康护理、个人照料和服务。

注:《现代汉语词典(第7版)》将"意"照护为照料护理。

2.2

老年照护师 elderly caregiver

经过老年照护知识和技能培训,了解老年人特点及相关的法律法规,熟悉老年医疗照护知识,掌握老年照护技能,经考试或考核取得合格证书的老年照护人员。

3 老年照护师分级

3.1 初级老年照护师:经过初级老年照护师培训并考核合格,具备老年基本照护技能和能力的照护人员。

3.2 中级老年照护师:经过中级老年照护师培训并考核合格,具备较高照护能力和较多照护经验的照护人员。

3.3 高级老年照护师:经过高级老年照护师培训并考核合格,具备全面照护能力和丰富照护经验的照护人员。

4 通用要求

4.1 应具有完全民事行为能力,无犯罪记录及不良从业记录。

4.2 应具有初中及以上学历,且年龄18岁~60岁。

4.3 应体检合格,持有二级及以上医疗机构出具的本人近3个月内的健康体检合格证明,无精神病史,无传染性疾病,无影响履行照护职责的疾病。

4.4 应具有职业责任和职业道德,关爱、尊重、理解、包容老年人。

4.5 应具有与老年人和家属有效的沟通能力,表达准确,解释耐心。

4.6 应定期参加老年照护师培训学习,取得由中国老年医学学会颁发的老年照护师等级证书。

5 基本职业要求

5.1 应了解掌握相关法律、法规,如老年人权益保障法,劳动法等。

5.2　应了解并掌握照护老人的应急预案,包括但不限于:消防安全、食品安全、设施设备安全、服务风险等。

5.3　应掌握基础急救技能,如心肺复苏术等。

5.4　应掌握老年日常生活照护技能,如进餐、排泄、洗漱、更衣、清洁、翻身、助行等,引导老年人参与康复和健康锻炼;负责与老年人交流沟通,协助实施心理健康计划及心理疏导。

5.5　应了解老年基本综合评估,能配合医疗护理人员进行主动观察、记录照护对象的身体状况,及时发现异常情况,并及时与专业人员沟通。

5.6　应熟悉老年常见病和慢性病的表现,了解基础医疗照护知识,为老年人提供基本生活照护、心理照护、饮食照护、服药照护、康复照护等服务。

5.7　应熟悉常见疾病的用药知识,了解被照护老人的用药物种类、名称、剂量和副作用,严格遵照医嘱协助老年人用药。

5.8　应熟悉居家常用医疗护理技术、家用医疗康复设备的使用方法。

5.9　应不断更新照护知识和技能,为照护对象提供更优质的服务。

6　技能要求

6.1　概述

本标准对初、中、高各级老年照护师的能力要求依次递进,高级别要求涵盖低级别。

6.2　初级老年照护师技能要求

6.2.1　符合 a)或 b):
   a)　应具有初中及以上学历证书,经过初级老年照护师培训考核合格者;
   b)　应具有护理专业中专及以上学历证书者。

6.2.2　掌握老年人基本照护技能,主要提供生活照料、基础护理,关注老年人基本营养需求,指导与协助老人身体活动:
   a)　应掌握老年人日常生活的照护技能,独立完成照护工作,如:协助老年人进餐、排泄、清洁、翻身、助行、陪伴等;
   b)　应掌握老年人因常见慢性疾病所致失能的照护技能,如:脑卒中患者恢复期的身体移动,协助老年人正确使用轮椅、拐杖等助行器,认知障碍老人生活照护等;
   c)　应掌握老年人常见安全问题及并发症预防的照护技能,如:预防跌倒、预防压疮等;
   d)　应掌握基本的老年用药知识,按照医嘱给老人服药,能阅读药物说明书,了解药物使用方法;
   e)　应掌握居家常用医疗仪器,如:血压计、制氧机等的使用方法,掌握常用家用电器、老年辅助用具等的使用方法;
   f)　应语言交流顺畅,能够理解、包容老年群体,特别是失能老人。

6.3　中级老年照护师技能要求

6.3.1　符合下列条件之一:
   a)　应取得初级老年照护师资格后从事老年照护工作 2 年及以上,经中级老年照护师培训考核合格者;
   b)　应具有初中及以上学历证书,实际从业老年照护工作 5 年及以上者;
   c)　应具有护理和相关专业中专及以上学历证书,且实际从事老年护理或照护工作 1 年以上者。

6.3.2　在 6.2.2 基础上增加急救基本能力、康复照护、健康指导等:
   a)　应掌握老年人常见健康问题及慢性疾病的急救处理,了解老年人常见疾病用药的种类、名称、剂量和主要副作用；

b) 应掌握老年人一般体能锻炼方法和康复训练方法；

c) 应掌握居家常用医疗仪器如:血糖仪、脉氧仪等的使用方法；

d) 应针对老年人的饮食习惯及健康要求,进行健康生活方式指导；

e) 应善于与老年人交流沟通,能有针对性地进行心理疏导；

f) 应能独立完成失能老年人的生活照护工作,如:鼻饲、口腔清洁等。

6.4 高级老年照护师技能要求

6.4.1 符合下列条件之一：

a) 取得中级老年照护师资格后从事老年照护工作 3 年及以上,经高级老年照护师培训考核合格者；

b) 具有护理和相关专业中专及以上学历证书,且实际从事老年护理或照护工作 2 年以上者。

6.4.2 在 6.3.2 基础上增加专科照护、风险防控、健康维护等：

a) 应能根据老年人的个体情况,完成科学、合理、有效的照护方案,提供优质的照护服务；

b) 应掌握老年人常见慢性病照护技术,如:排痰、吞咽功能障碍照护；

c) 应具备观察老年人病情变化的能力,且能向家属和医务人员清晰表达；

d) 应掌握老年人风险防控的照护技能,能够根据照护对象个体情况,完成预防跌倒、预防压疮等各种安全照护计划,掌握Ⅰ-Ⅱ级压疮的照护方法,协助老人进行体能锻炼、康复训练等；

e) 应掌握居家常用医疗仪器,如:排痰仪、雾化器等的使用方法；

f) 应协助实施心理健康计划；

g) 应能够制定科学合理、个性化的膳食方案,适应老年人的饮食习惯；

h) 应具备较强的学习能力,能够通过各种渠道学习和掌握新的照护知识与技能。

7 培训及考核

7.1 培训

7.1.1 应参加中国老年医学学会每年组织的老年照护师等级培训项目；

7.1.2 初级老年照护师培训不少于 480 个学时,中级老年照护师培训不少于 320 个学时,高级老年照护师培训不少于 160 个学时；

7.1.3 各级老年照护师取得合格证书后,每两年参加继续教育不少于 20 学时。

7.2 考核

7.2.1 经考试核合格的人员,颁发中国老年医学学会老年照护师等级证书。

7.2.2 老年照护师等级证书信息在中国老年医学学会指定网站发布。

7.2.3 获得老年照护师等级证书后,若有违法违规行为,将取消其所获证书资质并予以通报。

ICS 03.080
A 20

Social Organization Standard

T/CGSS 001—2018

Specification for elderly caregiver

老年照护师规范

（English Translation）

Issue date：2018-11-01   **Implementation date**：2018-11-01

Issued by Chinese Geriatrics Society

Foreword

This standard was drafted in accordance with the rules given in GB/T 1. 1—2009.

This standard was proposed by Geriatrics Medical Care Branch of Chinese Geriatrics Society.

This standard was prepared by Chinese Geriatrics Society.

This standard was drafted by Geriatrics Medical Care Branch of Chinese Geriatrics Society, Chinese PLA General Hospital, Peking Union Medical College Hospital, Beijing Geriatric Hospital, The First Affiliated Hospital of Zhejiang University, Army Medical University, Shengjing Hospital of Chinese Medical University, Changhai Hospital of the Second Military Medical University, Hunan Cancer Hospital, Zhujiang Hospital of Southern Medical University, West China Hospital Sichuan University, PLA Lanzhou General Hospital, Liaoning Province Jinqiu Hospital, PLA Northern Theatre Command General Hospital, The Affiliated Hospital of Medical School of Ningbo University, Chengdu Eighth People's Hospital, College of Psychology and Sociology of Shenzhen University, Qinggang Senior Care Center of the First Affiliated Hospital of Chongqing Medical University and Beijing Fengtai District Kangzhu Senior Care Center.

The main drafters of this standard were Hongying Pi, Huiru Hou, Na Guo, Baofeng Deng, Yanni Yang, Bing Zhu, Qin Zhang, Ling Fan, Lingjuan Zhang, Yongyi Chen, Xueqin Liu, Xiuying Hu, Hao Lu, Linshu Kong, Xuejun Hu, Zhiren Sheng, Jianli Hu, Qing Guan, Xiuli Yu, Anan Yu, Xiaoyuan Wang, Jing Yang, Haiyan Shi, Jing Sun, Chunyun Lai and Yuchun Liu.

Specification for elderly caregiver

1 Scope

This standard specifies the grade levels, general conditions, basic professional requirements, skill requirements, training and assessment of elderly caregivers.

The standard is applicable to the guidance for the training, grade evalution and assessment of elderly caregivers.

2 Terms and definitions

For the purposes of this document, the following terms and definitions apply.

2.1
elderly care

providing various services including basic health care and personal assistance for the elderly with partial or complete dysfunction.

Note: Care refers to providing care to and looking after someone in the *Contemporary Chinese Dictionary* (7th edition).

2.2
elderly caregiver

a professional who have received professional training and education in elderly care as well as relevant laws and regulations ,have equipped with the knowledge and skills of elderly care,have passed the qualification exams or assessment, and have been issued the elderly care certifications

3 Grade levels of elderly caregiver

3.1 Entry-level elderly caregivers are required to receive the minimum training to pass the entry-level qualification exams, and to have the basic elderly care skills and ability.

3.2 Intermediate-level elderly caregivers are required to receive additional training to pass the intermediate-level qualification exams and to have higher level of ability and experience in elderly care.

3.3 Advanced-level elderly caregivers are required to receive intensive training to pass the advanced-level qualification exams, and are expected to have deep ability and extensive experience in elderly care.

4 General conditions

4.1 Shall have full civil legal capacity. Shall have no criminal records or illegal employment records.

4.2 At least a junior high school diploma required for people aged from 18 to 60 years old.

4.3 Shall pass the physical examinations with the health certificate issued within 3 months by qualified medical institutions. Shall have no medical history of any mental illness, infectious disease or diseases and disabilities affecting work performance.

4.4 Shall have a strong professional responsibility and professional ethic. Shall demonstrate a high-level care for the elderly with kindness, respect, understanding and tolerance.

4.5 Shall communicate effectively and accurately with the elderly and their families , and explain patiently.

4.6 Shall participate regularly in elderly care training and hold the grade certificates of elderly caregiver issued by the Chinese Geriatrics Society.

5 Basic professional requirements

5.1 Understand and master related laws and regulations, such as *Law of the People's Republic of China on Protection of the Rights and Interests of the Elderly*, *Labor Law of the People's Republic of China*, etc.

5.2 Be able to react quickly in case of emergency, equipped with knowledge of but not limited to safety conducts of fire, food, equipment and devices, care provision related risks, etc.

5.3 Know how to perform first aid ,such as cardiopulmonary resuscitation (CPR).

5.4 Assist the elderly with their daily activities, such as feeding, toileting assistance, washing, dressing, bathing, grooming, changing bedridden patient's position, assisting in walking and daily movement, engage the elderly in physical exercise and physical therapy, and provide mental health and psychological care guidance.

5.5 Understand comprehensive geriatric health assessment, assist medical staff to actively make observations, keep medical and health records, and report any medical conditions to medical professionals in a timely manner.

5. 6 Recognize signs and symptoms of common diseases and chronic medical conditions of the elderly, and provide basic medical care in addition to daily care including psychological care, meal preparation, medication and rehabilitation assistance and other services.

5. 7 Understand the common usage of medications and help guide the elderly to adhere to medication treatments. Master knowledge of commonly used medications, category, name, dosage and side effects of the medications of the elderly and provide strict adherence plans under the doctor's instruction.

5. 8 Master common skills in homecare medicine and know how to use home medical equipment correctly.

5. 9 Conduct continuing education on updated knowledge and skills of elderly care to provide better services for customers.

6 Skill requirements

6. 1 Overview

The section provides guidelines for entry level, intermediate level and advanced level elderly caregivers and nursing staff. The required capability increases as the grade level increases.

6. 2 Entry-level elderly caregivers' requirements

6. 2. 1 a) or b):

a) At least a junior high school diploma required and pass the entry-level qualification exam,

b) At least a vocational nursing diploma required.

6. 2. 2 The entry-level elderly caregiver must have the basic elderly care skills, including assistance in daily care and providing nutrition guidance and physical exercise instructions.

a) Be able to independently provide daily care services feeding, toileting assistance, washing, dressing, bathing, grooming, changing bedridden patient's position, assisting in daily movement and walking and basic companionship, etc.).

b) Be able to provide specific care for the elderly with disabilities and chronic diseases, such as mobility assistance during stroke recovery, assistance with wheelchair and crutches, extensive care for the elderly with cognitive impairment,

c) Be able to adhere to safety standards and prevent common complications such as slip and fall and bedsores of bed-ridden elderly,

d) Be able to understand and follow the instructions of medication and help the elderly adhere to medication treatments,

e) Be able to use common home medical equipment and devices, such as sphygmomanometer, oxygen machine, as well as household appliances and elderly aid products,

f) Be able to communicate effectively with the elderly with respect and dignity, especially those with cognitive and physical disabilities.

6.3 Intermediate-level elderly caregivers' requirements

6.3.1 a) or b) or c):

a) Have been engaged in elderly care for 2 years or more after obtaining the qualification of entry-level elderly caregivers, and have passed the training and examination of intermediate-level elderly caregivers.

b) At least a junior high school diploma required and at least 5 years of elderly care work experience.

c) At least a vocational diploma in nursing or related field required and at least 1 year of elderly care experience.

6.3.2 Knowing how to perform first aid, rehabilitation nursing and health guidance ,etc. ,are required on the basis of 6.2.2.

a) Be able to identify and react properly to common health issue and chronic diseases of the elderly, be reactive in emergency, and have the knowledge of the types, names, dosage and main side effects of commonly used medications.

b) Be able to master the safety protections on physical fitness and rehabilitation training for the elderly.

c) Be able to use home medical equipment such as blood glucose meter and pulse oximeter.

d) Be able to provide a scientific guidance of healthy lifestyle for the elderly based on their dietary habits and health requirements.

e) Be good at communicating with the elderly and providing them targeted psychological counseling.

f) Be able to provide life assistance for the disabled elderly such as nasal feeding and oral hygiene.

6.4 Advanced-level elderly caregivers' requirements

6.4.1 a) or b):

a) Have been engaged in elderly care for 3 years or more after obtaining the qualification of intermediate-level elderly caregivers, and have passed the training and examination of advanced-level elderly caregivers.

b) Have a vocational diploma in nursing or related field with 2 years or more of elderly care work experience.

6.4.2 Advanced-level caregivers shall demonstrate specific health care capabilities, risk prevention and health maintenance on the basis of 6.3.2.

a) Be able to make scientific, reasonable and effective nursing plans according to the customer's medical condition and provide better services.

b) Provide nursing care for the elderly with common chronic conditions, such as sputum excretion and nursing of swallowing dysfunction.

c) Pay great attention to significant changes in the elderly and communicate promptly with family members and medical staff.

d) Be able to prevent the foreseeable risks in elderly care, for example, setting up preventive measures for slip and fall, making preventions on level one to two bedsore, and engaging the elderly in physical and rehabilitation exercise.

e) Be able to use home medical equipment such as airway clearance device and nebulizer.

f) Be good at communicating with the elderly and assisting them to engage in mental health care,

g) Be able to set up a proper and individual meal schedule based on the client's dietary habits.

h) Be able to learn , adapt and conduct continuing education through different channels and master new knowledge and skills in elderly care field.

7 Training and assessment

7.1 Training

7.1.1 The training program is provided yearly by Chinese geriatrics society.

7.1.2 The elderly caregivers shall attend the training program of Chinese geriatrics society. The entry-level caregivers must have at least 480 hours of in-class training, the intermediate-level caregivers shall have at least 320 hours of in-class training, and the advanced-level caregivers must have at least 160 hours of in-class training.

7.1.3 The caregivers shall continue to have at least 20 hours of in-class training every other year after obtaining the certification.

7.2 Assessment

7.2.1 Those who have passed the examination or assessment will be awarded the grade certificate of elderly caregiver issued by Chinese geriatrics society.

7.2.2 The information of certificate of elderly caregiver will be released on the official website of the Chinese geriatrics society.

7.2.3 The elderly caregiver certificate will be suspended upon any criminal misconduct of the certification holder.

———————————

ICS 03.080
A 20

团 体 标 准

T/CGSS 003—2019

老年友善服务规范

Specification for age-friendly service

2019-03-01 发布   2019-03-01 实施

中国老年医学学会　发 布

前　言

本标准按照 GB/T 1.1—2009 给出的规则起草。

本标准由北京老年医院提出。

本标准由中国老年医学学会归口。

本标准起草单位:北京老年医院、中国老年医学学会老年医疗机构管理分会、北京医联老年医学培训与咨询中心、辽宁省老年病医院(辽宁省金秋医院)、郑州市老年病医院(郑州市第九人民医院)、江苏省老年医院、河北省老年病医院、海南省老年医院、成都市第八人民医院、成都市老年康疗院、四川省自贡市第五人民医院、乐山老年病专科医院、云南省康复医院(昆明市老年病医院)、国药东风花果医院、内蒙古科尔沁区老年医院、淄博淄建集团医院、大庆油田东海医院、唐山工人集团医院、太原市第二人民医院、北京市东城区中西医结合老年病医院。

本标准主要起草人:宋岳涛、陈峥、张进平、刘霜秋、宋惠平、李保英、暴继敏、白建林、许家仁、刘建军、金水晶、毕卫红、彭代之、肖洪松、谭友果、朱斌、田福建、胡万保、牟晓红、邓小蕴、张春林、李玉杰、卢艳丽。

老年友善服务规范

1 范围

本标准规定了老年友善服务的基本要求、服务内容与要求、服务评价及改进。
本标准适用于提供老年友善服务的医疗、康复、护理和照护等服务机构。

2 规范性引用文件

下列文件对于本文件的应用是必不可少的。凡是注日期的引用文件,仅注日期的版本适用于本文件。凡是不注日期的引用文件,其最新版本(包括所有的修改单)适用于本文件。

GB/T 16432 康复辅助器具 分类和术语
GB/T 17242 投诉处理指南
T/CGSS 001 老年照护师规范

3 术语和定义

GB/T 16432 界定的以及下列术语和定义适用于本文件。

3.1
老年友善服务 age-friendly service
为老年人营造尊重、关爱与支持的环境,开展能够满足其特殊需求并符合其身心特点的医疗、康复、护理和照护等活动。

3.2
老年综合评估 comprehensive geriatric assessment
由多学科专业人员为功能下降、衰弱的老年人从体能、认知、心理、社会、环境和疾病等多方面进行全面评估的健康测量方法。

3.3
多学科整合管理 inter-disciplinary integrated management
由老年病医师、康复医师与康复治疗师、护师(士)、心理师、营养师、临床药师、个案管理师和社会工作者等构成的多学科团队,依据老年综合评估的结果对老年患者实施综合性的医疗、康复和护理服务的模式。

3.4
老年综合征 geriatric syndrome,GS
由多种慢性病的病理过程或多种诱发因素导致的具有同一临床表现特点的老年病征。

4 基本要求

4.1 服务机构

4.1.1 服务机构包括医院、康复院、护理院、养老院及提供医养结合服务的养老照护中心等。

4.1.2 应依法登记注册。

4.1.3 应有为老人服务的管理部门和专职人员,有组织管理的制度、流程、服务规范和应急预案。

4.1.4 应建立老年友善服务中不良事件的上报与处理反馈管理系统,宜参照《全国医院信息化建设标准与规范(试行)》。

4.1.5 应有负责双向转诊服务的管理部门和专职人员。

4.1.6 应对服务人员进行岗前、岗中安全知识与技能的培训,培训时数每年均不少于 20 学时,培训考核达标后方能上岗。

4.1.7 宜单独设立或合作建立老年人长期照护病区或老年护理院,参照《护理院基本标准》执行。

4.1.8 宜建立社会工作部、志愿者部等组织机构和管理制度,有长期招募志愿者特别是老年志愿者的计划。

4.1.9 应妥善保管各种服务的原始文档,实现服务全程留痕,责任可追溯。

4.2 服务人员

4.2.1 应提供身体健康证明,具备良好的职业道德,尊重老年人的民族习俗和宗教信仰,注意保护其个人隐私和信息安全。

4.2.2 应具备与老年人良好沟通能力。对失能、失智的老年人使用慢速、清晰的语言,或采用肢体语言、文字或图片进行交流。支持和鼓励参与老年人的健康管理。

4.2.3 专业技术服务人员应具备相关资质,参加相关培训,熟练掌握本岗位设施设备的安全使用规程和卫生清洁要求。

4.2.4 医疗、医技服务人员应掌握常见老年疾病诊疗技术、老年综合评估技术、老年综合征风险筛查与干预技术,定期为老年人开展义诊、疾病筛查和健康宣教活动。

4.2.5 护理人员应熟练掌握老年综合评估技术,依据评估结果制定个性化的护理计划;应具备向老年人或者监护人提供适合居家、社区或机构养老,或者入院治疗的判断与建议的老年护理及管理能力。

4.2.6 老年医学科及相关医学科室科主任应具有老年医学教育或培训达标的副主任医师以上职称;护理负责人应具有老年护理专业的主管护师以上职称。

4.2.7 康复治疗师应具有中级及以上专业技术职称。康复治疗科室负责人应具有中级及以上专业技术职称并从事康复治疗工作 5 年以上。

4.2.8 老年用药与营养咨询门诊的医师或护师应由有 5 年以上相关临床经验。

4.2.9 老年照护师应符合 T/CGSS 001 要求。

4.3 服务机构环境与设施

4.3.1 场所应适合老年人生理、病理特点和功能状况,为失能、失智老年人提供移动、如厕等无障碍环境,以安全、便捷为基本要求。

4.3.2 应配置适老辅具设施;公示的服务信息应置于明显位置,并便于老年人阅读和理解。

4.3.3 服务机构的整体环境、病房环境、卫生间和浴室环境、通道和电梯环境、交通设施和标识系统宜达到老年友善服务环境与设施条件。参见表 A.1。

5 服务内容与要求

5.1 老年综合评估

5.1.1 应对服务机构内的老年人开展老年综合评估服务,评估内容及评估方法见表 1。

表 1　老年综合评估内容与方法

序号	评估内容	评估表或评估工具
1	一般医学评估	包括患病与用药情况的评估,参见表 B.1
2	日常生活活动能力评估	基本日常生活活动能力评估量表(Barthel 指数),参见表 B.2
3	平衡功能评估	平衡试验,参见表 B.3
		前臂伸展试验,参见表 B.4
4	认知功能评估	简易认知评估工具(Mini-Cog),参见表 B.5
		简易智能评估量表(MMSE),参见表 B.6
5	视力评估	视力简易评估法,参见表 B.7
6	听力评估	听力简易评估法,参见表 B.8
7	社会评估	社会参与功能简易评估法(见民政部《老年人能力评估标准》),参见表 B.9
8	居家安全评估	家庭危险因素评估工具(HFHA),参见表 B.10

5.1.2　评估人员应根据评估结果提出具有针对性的干预措施,必要时经过多学科小组共同讨论和制定干预方案。

5.1.3　宜对出院回家的老年患者,进行居家安全的评估与提供居家环境适老化改造建议。居家安全的评估应包括对灯光、地面、卫生间、厨房、客厅、卧室、走廊或过道等的评估,家庭危险因素评估工具(HF-HA)参见表 B.10。

5.1.4　应将评估结果录入病历或服务档案,并进行数据的分析、管理与应用。

5.2　老年综合征和老年照护问题的评估与干预

5.2.1　老年综合征包括跌倒、痴呆、谵妄、衰弱、肌少症、多重用药、抑郁、晕厥、尿失禁、帕金森综合征、便秘、睡眠障碍和慢性疼痛等。老年照护问题包括深静脉血栓、肺栓塞、压疮、骨质疏松与骨折、吸入性肺炎等。

5.2.2　应开展对老年综合征和老年照护问题的评估。老年综合征和老年照护问题的评估见表 2。

5.2.3　服务机构应根据老年综合征和老年照护问题的评估结果,提出并实施具有针对性的干预措施,如制定并实施老年跌倒风险防控或跌倒损伤的救治措施,制定并实施防治老年痴呆、老年谵妄和老年抑郁的干预措施,为营养不良者出具营养和运动处方,为长期卧床的老年患者进行压疮风险的防控或为已发生压疮者实施正确有效的治疗和护理。

5.2.4　对老年综合征和老年照护问题的干预措施应有效果评价。

表 2　老年综合征和老年照护问题的评估内容

序号	评估内容	评估表
1	跌倒评估	跌倒风险评估量表,参见表 B.11
		Morse 跌倒评估量表,参见表 B.12
2	痴呆评估	简易智能评估量表(MMSE),参见表 B.6
		临床痴呆量表(CDR),参见表 B.13
3	谵妄评估	老年谵妄评估法(CAM),参见表 B.14
4	营养不良评估	微型营养评定法(MNA),参见表 B.15
		营养风险筛查法(NRS2002),参见表 B.16
5	抑郁评估	老年抑郁评估量表简表(GDS-5),参见表 B.17
		老年抑郁评估量表(GDS-15),参见表 B.18
6	压疮评估	皮肤危险因子评估表(Braden 量表),参见表 B.19

5.3 老年人高风险状态检测及处置

5.3.1 应针对老年人跌倒、坠床、窒息、肺栓塞等高风险指标进行监测与识别,除应对患者、家属及照护人员做出风险告知外,还应有风险标识和其他相应的防范措施。

5.3.2 应制定急性脑卒中、急性心肌梗死、高血压危象、心力衰竭、呼吸衰竭和肾衰竭的应急抢救措施。

5.4 常见老年病的防控

5.4.1 常见老年疾病主要包括但不限于高血压、糖尿病、高血脂症、脑卒中、冠心病、慢性阻塞性肺疾病、肺部感染、关节病变、晚期肿瘤和慢性肾病等疾病。

5.4.2 应开展对老年人群慢性病综合防控,对高风险人群采取运动与营养等干预方式。应有具体活动记录,包括活动通知、活动主题、主办方、受众人数及现场视频或照片等。

5.4.3 宜设立常见老年疾病的健康教育科普宣传场地,并有专、兼职人员负责制定活动计划、组织实施和进行活动情况的记录。机构内宜配备有宣教器材和投放设备,并能够保持正常使用。

5.5 老年人用药评估

5.5.1 应对老年人用药进行全面评估(参见表 B.1),并对不合理用药进行指导。

5.5.2 在老年患者离开机构时,应告知用药注意事项。

5.6 多学科整合管理

5.6.1 根据需要对病情复杂、多重用药、多系统功能障碍、多脏器衰竭的老年患者进行多学科整合管理服务。

5.6.2 应有多学科小组会议的讨论记录,有为老年患者形成的整合管理方案和预防其并发症发生的处理意见。

5.6.3 医护人员应鼓励老年患者及其家属参与多学科小组会议,并参与相关活动。

5.7 老年医学专科服务

5.7.1 宜为老年患者提供老年综合征、脑卒中、认知障碍、骨性关节病、老年跌倒、睡眠障碍、压疮、精神疾患等的医疗照护与康复服务。

5.7.2 宜为老年人开展营养干预服务,根据营养风险评估结果开展营养知识教育和提供营养处方。

5.7.3 宜对老年患者开展中期照护、长期照护和安宁疗护等服务。

5.7.4 宜为老年人开展居家适老环境评估和适老辅具适配等服务,参照《中国康复辅助器具目录》进行配置。

5.7.5 老年专科服务应有病历和服务记录。

5.8 延伸服务

5.8.1 延伸服务是指机构依据出院计划为回到社区或居家的老年人继续提供医疗、护理、功能康复和社会支持等延续性的服务。主要服务内容与要求见表3。

表 3　主要延伸服务内容与要求

序号	服务内容	服务要求
1	延续性照护计划	应至少包括健康宣教、日常生活能力恢复训练、饮食指导、运动干预、高血压和糖尿病等慢性疾病的管理等服务
2	双向转诊服务	应由负责双向转诊服务的管理部门和专职人员为老年患者提供评估后的转诊服务
3	复诊服务	应由医院门诊或宜由网络门诊为老年患者提供预约复诊服务
4	绿色通道	应在挂号、交费、候诊、取药、检查等窗口为特殊情况的老年人开设就医绿色通道
5	健康管理	应为居家签约、养老机构或其他长期照护机构中的老年人建立健康档案和服务档案
6	技术指导	应为周边社区卫生服务机构或养老机构中的医护人员提供现场技术指导或远程医学服务

5.8.2　延伸服务应有服务记录和效果评估。

6　服务评价及改进

6.1　服务评价

6.1.1　评价内容包括本标准第 4 章和第 5 章的内容。

6.1.2　服务评价包括：服务机构自我评价、服务对象评价和第三方评价。

——服务机构自我评价应根据服务内容及服务要求定期进行自我评价。

——服务机构应定期开展服务对象的满意度评价。

——中国老年医学学会可委托具有资质的第三方机构开展老年友善服务的评价。

6.2　改进

6.2.1　服务机构应根据评价结果，对不符合要求的项目制定整改方案，跟踪实施，及时改进，不断提高服务质量。

6.2.2　在服务过程中随时收集有关服务质量问题信息，分析原因，制定纠正措施，对过程或管理进行整改，避免再次发生。

6.2.3　服务机构应主动接受社会监督，对外公布监督和投诉电话、投诉方法、投诉流程，建立服务质量投诉及纠纷处理、反馈机制，应按照 GB/T 17242 的要求处理投诉事件。

附　录　A
（资料性附录）
老年友善服务环境与设施

老年友善服务环境与设施见表 A.1。

表 A.1　老年友善服务环境与设施

序号	项目	老年友善服务环境与设施
1	整体环境	整体环境保持清洁舒适和安全
		地板、墙壁、家具宜用暖色；房门、扶手宜用高对比颜色区分；地板材料无反光、防滑，不宜用夸张的几何图案和斑纹
		通风系统无噪声，通风良好
		电动门自动阻尼延时≥4 s
2	病房	病房照明均匀充足、无眩光；设置有夜灯
		病房及公共区域窗户安装行程限位装置
		床间距留有轮椅转弯半径空间；病床高度以患者小腿长度 100%～120% 为宜（坐时双脚踏实着地）；床挡高度以高出褥垫 350 mm 为宜；长期卧床者宜用减压床垫和座椅垫
		床边安装呼叫器，按钮方便触及；床边宜有清晰易于使用的床灯开关
		病房内宜装有大字静音时钟和日历，高风险病患床边要有标识
3	卫生间和浴室	卫生间采用坐便式马桶，轮椅或移行装置与马桶零距离（每病区最低配置 1～2 间）；门诊等公共区域宜设无障碍、无性别厕所
		坐便器临空侧设固定式或上翻式扶手，扶手距坐便器中心线水平距离 350 mm～400 mm，放下时上层扶手距地高度 700 mm；临墙侧设 L 形扶手，坐便器中心线距墙面 450 mm，L 形扶手垂直段距坐便器前沿 200 mm～250 mm，最高点距地 1 400 mm 以上，水平段距地 700 mm
		坐便器双侧宜安装输液挂钩；宜在侧前方墙面安装呼叫按钮或拉绳式呼叫装置，按钮中心距地面高度 400 mm～500 mm，拉绳下垂末端距地 100 mm，以便于触摸。宜有专岗随时接收呼叫信号并开展施救
		卫生间门宽≥900 mm，宜双向或推拉开门；洗手盆下方净高不宜＜650 mm，方便轮椅出入
		病区宜设置公共浴室或配备可供自理、半自理、不能自理病人洗浴的设施和设备；使用轮椅患者的浴室宜留有轮椅转弯半径空间；淋浴区要有马桶或坐便椅，浴缸或淋浴花洒下应有防滑垫；洗澡/淋浴开关高度宜考虑坐轮椅者使用方便
		马桶、小便池、淋浴和浴缸侧面应安装上推式或 L 型高度适中的扶手
4	家具、扶手、通道、电梯	床头柜如有轮子应是制动脚轮；家具锐角宜做钝角处理；餐桌高度以轮椅进出顺畅为宜；座椅要有扶手、软垫，防滑，易清洁，高度以坐者双脚掌完全着地为宜
		宜在楼梯和走廊墙体侧安装扶手，坡道至少一侧有扶手，楼梯扶手长度宜超出坡道和楼梯的两端；并在终端 100 mm 处有结束提醒
		坡道高度与长度适宜比为 1∶20；坡道长度超过 9 m 宜设休息平台

表 A.1（续）

序号	项目	老年友善服务环境与设施
4	家具、扶手、通道、电梯	>50 m 的长走道和楼梯拐角要设有休息区或休息椅
		走道、坡道宽度能使两个轮椅并行通过,地面无高差,避免轮椅、拐杖等卡住
		坡道和楼梯两端地面要有清晰可辨的起始和结束的提示标识
		在未设专人开关电梯服务的电梯内外,呼叫按钮应用醒目的颜色和字体;电梯门开关阻尼延时≥4 s;电梯轿厢宜三面安装扶手
5	交通设施	医院门诊和住院病区主出入口宜设有无障碍通道,主入口处有方便老年人上、下车的临时停车区或车位
		台阶、坡道、转弯处宜有安全警示标志和标识,如限速、禁止鸣笛、急转弯、减速
		医院门急诊、住院病区宜有移乘设备(如轮椅、平车等)可供患者使用
6	标识系统	医院院区内主要道路岔口、建筑主出入口及各楼层均宜设有颜色对比明显的导向标志;标识保持颜色、字体和材质统一,导引图上要标明当前位置
		标识应使用简单易懂的语言,配合简单的图形;小标识牌字体大小至少 40 mm,大标识牌字体至少 60 mm
		坡道和楼梯两端地面要有清晰可辨的起始和结束的提示标识

附　录　B
（资料性附录）
老年综合评估量表

老年综合评估量表见表 B.1～B.19。

表 B.1　一般医学评估

序号	评估内容	评估结果		
1	患病情况评估	1. 4. 7. 10.	2. 5. 8. 11.	3. 6. 9. 12.
2	用药情况评估	1. 4. 7. 10.	2. 5. 8. 11.	3. 6. 9. 12.

表 B.2　基本日常生活活动能力评估量表（Barthel 指数）

序号	项目	填表说明	评分	得分
1	大便控制（排便）	指 1 周内情况 偶尔＝1 周 1 次	0 分＝完全失控 5 分＝偶尔失控（每周≤1 次），或需要他人提示 10 分＝可控制大便	
2	小便控制（排尿）	指 24 h～48 h 情况 "偶尔"指≤1 次/天	0 分＝完全失控，或留置导尿管 5 分＝偶尔失控（每天≤1 次，每周＞1 次），或需要他人提示 10 分＝可控制小便或插尿管的病人能独立完成尿管的放开与关闭	
3	修饰（指洗脸、刷牙、梳头、刮脸等）	指 24 h～48 h 情况	0 分＝需他人帮助 5 分＝可自己独立完成，或由看护者提供工具：如挤好牙膏，准备好水等	
4	如厕（包括去厕所、解开衣裤、擦净、整理衣裤、冲水）	患者应能独立完成如厕的全过程	0 分＝需极大帮助或完全依赖他人 5 分＝需部分帮助（需他人搀扶去厕所、需他人帮忙冲水或整理衣裤等） 10 分＝可独立完成	
5	进食（指用餐具将食物由容器送到口中、咀嚼、吞咽等过程）	患者应能独立完成进食全过程，食物可由其他人做或端来	0 分＝需极大帮助或完全依赖他人，或有留置营养管 5 分＝需部分帮助（进食需要一定帮助，如协助把持餐具、夹菜、盛饭） 10 分＝可独立进食（在合理的时间内独立进食准备好的食物）	

表 B.2（续）

序号	项目	填表说明	评分	得分
6	移位（床椅转移）	指从床到椅子，然后回来	0分＝完全依赖他人，不能坐 5分＝需极大帮助（2人）、能坐（较大程度上依赖他人搀扶和帮助） 10分＝需部分帮助（1人）或指导（需他人搀扶或使用拐杖） 15分＝可独立完成	
7	平地行走（步行）	指在院内、屋内活动，可以借助辅助工具。如果用轮椅，应能拐弯或自行出门而不需帮助	0分＝完全依赖他人 5分＝需极大帮助（因肢体残疾、平衡能力差、过度衰弱、视力等问题，在较大程度上依赖他人搀扶，或坐在轮椅上自行移动） 10分＝需部分帮助（因肢体残疾、平衡能力差、过度衰弱、视力等问题，在一定程度上需他人的搀扶或使用拐杖、助行器等辅助用具） 15分＝可独立在平地上行走45 m	
8	穿衣（指穿脱衣服、系扣、拉拉链、穿脱鞋袜、系鞋带）	能独立完成穿衣动作	0分＝需极大帮助或完全依赖他人 5分＝需部分帮助（能自己穿脱，但需他人帮助整理衣物） 10分＝可独立完成（系开纽扣、拉链、穿鞋等）	
9	上下楼梯		0分＝不能 5分＝需帮助（体力或语言指导） 10＝自理（可独立借助辅助工具）	
10	洗澡	开关水龙头和调试水温，涂抹浴液和冲净等洗浴动作	0分＝依赖他人 5分＝自理	

评估总得分＿＿＿＿＿＿＿

评价标准：100分，能力完好；65分～95分，轻度受损；45分～60分，中度受损；≤40分，重度受损。

说明：总分为100分，得分越高，独立性越好，依赖性越小。

表 B.3 平衡试验

序号	试验方法	评估方法	站立时间/s
1	并足站立	两足紧贴并行站立	
2	半足距站立	两足紧贴差半足站立	
3	全足距站立	两足前后站成一条直线，前一足的足跟紧贴后一足的足尖	

评价标准：全足距站立时间≤10 s，说明平衡功能差，有跌倒的风险。

表 B.4　前臂伸展试验

试验方法	三次测量平均值	功能评价结果
第一步:患者肩靠墙壁站直,保持稳定状态,上肢向前平伸, 　　掌心向下握拳,尽量将拳头前伸	≤12 cm	平衡功能极差,跌倒风险大
	<15 cm	平衡性较差,有跌倒风险
第二步:以第三掌骨头的位置为测量起点,测量 3 次,取平均 　　值。评估时应预防病人跌倒	20～25 cm	平衡功能尚好
	≥25 cm	平衡功能良好

注:正常值为≥15 cm。

表 B.5　简易认知评估量表(Mini-Cog)

测试顺次	测试内容与结果	评分	得分
引导语	A."我说 3 样东西:苹果/手表/国旗.请重复一遍并记住,一会儿再问您"。 B.画钟测验:"请在这儿画一个圆形时钟,在时钟上标出 11 点 10 分"。 C.回忆词语:"现在请您告诉我,刚才我要您记住的 3 样东西是什么?"		
回答情况	____、____、____(不必按顺序)		
测试结果	画钟正确(画出一个闭锁圆,指针位置准确),且能回忆出 3 个词	3 分	
	画钟正确(画出一个闭锁圆,指针位置准确),且能回忆出 1～2 个词	2 分	
	画钟错误(画的圆不闭锁,或指针位置不准确),或只回忆出 1～2 个词	1 分	
	1 个词也回忆不出,已确诊为认知障碍,如老年痴呆	0 分	

评价标准:2～3 分,无失智;1 分,可疑失智;0 分:失智。

表 B.6　简易智能评估量表(MMSE)

检查项目	问题序号	评估项目	评分	得分
时间定向力	1	今年是哪一年?	答对 1 分,答错或拒答 0 分	
	2	现在是什么季节?	同上	
	3	现在是几月份?	同上	
	4	今天是几号?	同上	
	5	今天是星期几?	同上	
地点定向力	6	这是什么城市(名)?	同上	
	7	这是什么区(城区名)?	同上	
	8	这是什么医院(医院名或胡同名)?	同上	
	9	这是第几层楼?	同上	
	10	这是什么地方(地址、门牌号)?	同上	

引导语:现在我告诉您 3 种东西的名称,我说完后请您重复一遍。请您记住这 3 种东西:皮球、国旗和树木,过一会儿我还要问您(每样东西回答用时 1 s)。

记忆力	11	复述:皮球	同上	
	12	复述:国旗	同上	
	13	复述:树木	同上	

表 B.6（续）

检查项目	问题序号	评估项目	评分	得分
		引导语：现在请您做 100 减 7 的连续计算，请您将每减 1 个 7 后的答案告诉我，直到我说"停"为止。		
注意力和计算力	14	计算 100－7＝？	答对给 1 分，答错为 0 分	
	15	再次运算	答对给 1 分，答错为 0 分	
	16	再次运算	答对给 1 分，答错为 0 分	
	17	再次运算	答对给 1 分，答错为 0 分	
	18	再次运算	答对给 1 分，答错为 0 分	
		备注：如前一项计算错误，但在错误得数基础上减 7 正确者仍给相应得分		
		引导语：现在请您说出刚才我让您记住的是哪 3 种东西？		
回忆力	19	回忆：皮球	答对 1 分，答错或拒答 0 分	
	20	回忆：国旗	同上	
	21	回忆：树木	同上	
	22	检查者出示手表问受试者这是什么？	同上	
	23	检查者出示铅笔问受试者这是什么？	同上	
	24	请您跟我说"44 只石狮子"	能正确说出 1 分，否则 0 分	
	25	检查者给受试者一张卡片，上面写着"请闭上您的眼睛"请受试者念一念这句话，并按上面的意思去做	能正确说出并能做到 1 分，不正确说出，也不能做到 0 分	
		引导语：我给您一张纸，请您按我说的去做。现在开始，用右手拿着这张纸，用两只手把它对折起来，然后将它放在您的左腿上。		
语言能力	26	用右手拿着这张纸	正确给 1 分，错误给 0 分	
	27	用两只手将纸对折	能对折 1 分，不能为 0 分	
	28	将纸放在左腿上	放对给 1 分，答错为 0 分	
	29	请您写一个完整的句子	能正确写为 1 分，答错为 0 分	
	30	请您照着下面图案样子把它画下来	正确为 1 分，错误为 0 分	

评估总得分＿＿＿＿＿＿＿

说明：总分范围 0～30 分，正常与不正常的分界值与受教育程度有关：文盲（未受教育）组 17 分；小学（受教育年限 ≤6 年）组 20 分；中学或以上（受教育年限＞6 年）组 24 分。分界值以下为有认知功能缺陷，以上为正常。

表 B.7 视力简易评估表

序号	测试内容	评分	得分
1	能看清书报上的标准字体	4	
2	能看清楚大字体,但看不清书报上的标准字体	3	
3	视力有限,看不清报纸大标题,但能辨认物体	2	
4	辨认物体有困难,但眼睛能跟随物体移动,只能看到光、颜色和形状	1	
5	没有视力,眼睛不能跟随物体移动	0	

评估总得分 _____

说明:被测试者若平日戴老花镜或近视镜,可在佩戴眼镜的情况下进行测试。

推荐评价标准:4分,视力正常;3分,低视力;1~2分,盲;0分,完全失明。

表 B.8 听力简易评估表

序号	测试问题	评分	得分
1	可正常交谈,能听到电视、电话、门铃的声音	4	
2	在轻声说话或说话距离超过 2 m 时听不清	3	
3	正常交流有些困难,需在安静环境或大声说话才能听到	2	
4	讲话者大声说话或说话很慢,才能部分听见	1	
5	完全听不见	0	

说明:被测试者若平时佩戴助听器,可在佩戴助听器的情况下进行测试。

推荐评价标准:4分,听力正常;3分,听力下降;1~2分,听力障碍;0分,完全失聪。

表 B.9 社会参与功能简易评估法

序号	评估内容	评分	得分
1	参与社会,对社会环境有一定的适应能力,待人接物恰当	4	
2	能适应单纯环境,主动接触人,初见面时难让人发现智力问题,不能理解隐喻语	3	
3	脱离社会,可被动接触,不会主动待人,谈话中有很多不适词句,容易上当受骗	2	
4	勉强可与人交往,谈吐内容不清楚,表情不恰当	1	
5	难以与人接触	0	

评价标准:4分,能力完好;3分,轻度降低;2分:中度降低;0~1分:重度降低。

表 B.10　家庭危险因素评估工具（HFHA）及建议

评估项目	评估排序	评估内容	结果		建议
室内灯光	1	居室灯光是否合适	□是	□否	灯光不宜过亮或过暗
	2	楼道与台阶的灯光是否明亮	□是	□否	在通道和楼梯处使用 60 W 的灯泡。通道上宜装有光电效应的电灯
	3	电灯开关是否容易打开	□是	□否	应轻松开关电灯
	4	在床上是否容易开灯	□是	□否	在床上应很容易开灯
	5	存放物品的地方是否明亮	□是	□否	在黑暗处应安装灯泡。从亮处到暗处应稍候片刻
地面（板）	6	地面是否平整	□是	□否	地面不宜高低不平，如有应以斜坡代替。室内不应有门槛
	7	地毯（垫）是否平放，没有皱褶和边缘卷曲	□是	□否	确保地毯（垫）保持良好状态，去除破旧或卷曲的地毯
	8	地板的光滑度和软硬度是否合适	□是	□否	地面（板）不宜光滑，可以刷防滑的油漆，可铺地毯
	9	地板垫子是否无滑动	□是	□否	除去所有松动的地垫，或者将他们牢牢固定在地上，并且贴上防滑地衬垫
	10	一有溢出液体是否立即抹干	□是	□否	一有溢出的液体立即将其擦干净
	11	地面上是否放置杂乱的东西	□是	□否	地面上应整洁，尽可能不放或少放东西，应清除走廊障碍物
	12	通道上是否有电线	□是	□否	通道上不应有任何电线
卫生间	13	在浴缸或浴室内是否使用防滑垫	□是	□否	在湿的地面易滑倒，浴室内应使用防滑垫，在浴缸内也应使用防滑材料
	14	洗刷用品是否放在容易拿到的地方	□是	□否	洗刷用品应放在容易拿到的地方，以免弯腰或伸得太远
	15	在马桶周围、浴缸或淋浴间是否有扶手	□是	□否	应装合适的扶手
	16	是否容易在马桶上坐下和站起来	□是	□否	如马桶过低，或老人不易坐下和站起来，应加用马桶增高垫，并在周围装上合适的扶手
	17	浴缸是否过高	□是	□否	浴缸不宜过高。如过高，应加用洗澡凳或洗澡椅等
厨房	18	是否不用攀爬、弯腰或影响自己的平衡就可很容易取到常用的厨房用品	□是	□否	整理好厨房，以便能更容易取到最常用的厨具。可配用手推托盘车。如必须上高处取物，请用宽底座和牢靠的梯子
	19	厨房内灯光是否明亮	□是	□否	灯光应明亮
	20	是否常将溢出的液体立刻抹干净	□是	□否	应随时将溢出的液体抹干净

表 B.10（续）

评估项目	评估排序	评估内容	结果		建议
客厅	21	是否有良好的通风设备来减少眼睛变模糊的危险性	□是	□否	留置通风口,安装厨房抽油烟机或排气扇,做饭时更应通风
	22	是否有烟雾的报警装置	□是	□否	应装烟雾报警装置
	23	是否有家用灭火器	□是	□否	应配家用灭火器
	24	是否很容易从沙发椅上站起来	□是	□否	宜用高度适宜又有坚固扶手的椅子
	25	过道上是否放置有任何电线、家具和凌乱的东西	□是	□否	不可在过道上放置电话线、电线和其他杂物
	26	家具是否放置在合适的位置,使开窗或取物时不用把手伸得太远或弯腰	□是	□否	家具应放置在合适的位置,地面应平整、防滑和安全
卧室	27	窗帘等物品的颜色是否与周围环境太相近	□是	□否	窗帘等物品的颜色尽可能鲜艳,与周围环境应有明显区别
	28	室内是否有安全隐患,如过高或过低的椅子、杂乱的家居物品等	□是	□否	卧室的地板上不要放东西。要把卧室内松动的电话线和电线系好,通道上不得有杂乱物品。椅子高度应合适
	29	室内有无夜间照明设施? 是否可以在下床前开灯	□是	□否	床边安一盏灯,考虑按钮灯或夜明灯。夜晚最好在床边放一把手电筒
	30	室内有无紧急呼叫设施	□是	□否	安装紧急呼叫器
	31	是否容易上、下床	□是	□否	床高度应适中,较硬的床垫可方便上、下床。下床应慢,先坐起再缓慢站立
	32	卧室内是否有电话	□是	□否	卧室内应装部电话或接分机,放在在床上就可以够着的地方
	33	电热毯线是否已安全系好,不会使您绊倒? 按钮是否可在床上够得着	□是	□否	应将线系好,按钮应装在床上就可够得着的位置
	34	床罩是否有绳圈做的穗	□是	□否	床罩上不应有穗或绳等
	35	如果使用拐杖或助行器,它们是否放在下床前很容易够得着的地方	□是	□否	将拐杖或助行器放在较合适的地方
楼梯与梯子	36	是否能清楚地看见楼梯的边缘	□是	□否	楼梯与台阶处需要额外的照明,并应明亮。楼梯灯尽量使用自动开关
	37	楼梯与台阶的灯光是否明亮	□是	□否	灯光要明亮
	38	楼梯上、下是否有电灯开关	□是	□否	楼梯上、下要有电灯开关
	39	每一级楼梯的边缘是否安装防滑踏脚	□是	□否	在所有楼梯上必须至少一边有扶手,每一级楼梯的边缘应装防滑踏脚

表 B.10（续）

评估项目	评估排序	评估内容	结果		建议
	40	楼梯的扶手是否坚固	□是	□否	扶手必须坚固
	41	折梯和梯凳是否短而稳固,且梯脚装上防滑胶套	□是	□否	尽量避免使用梯子,如需用时最好有人在旁。折梯应保持良好状态,最好用有扶手的梯子,保证安全
衣服与鞋子	42	是否穿有防滑鞋底的鞋子	□是	□否	鞋子或拖鞋上应有防滑鞋底和凸出的纹路
	43	鞋子是否有宽大的鞋跟	□是	□否	鞋子上应有圆形宽大的鞋跟
	44	在房屋以外的地方是否穿的是上街的鞋子而不是拖鞋	□是	□否	避免只穿袜子、宽松的拖鞋、平底或其他滑溜鞋底的鞋子和高跟鞋
	45	穿的衣服是否合身和没有悬垂的绳子或褶边	□是	□否	衣服不宜太长,以免绊倒(尤其是睡衣)
	46	是否坐着穿衣	□是	□否	穿衣应坐下,而不要一条腿站立
住房外环境	47	阶梯的边缘是否已清楚标明	□是	□否	应在阶梯的前沿漆上不同的颜色确保所有外面的阶梯极易看到
	48	阶梯的边缘是否有自粘的防滑条	□是	□否	阶梯边缘应贴上防滑踏脚
	49	阶梯是否有牢固且容易抓的扶手	□是	□否	阶梯应有牢固且容易抓的扶手
	50	房子周围的小路情况是否良好	□是	□否	应保持小路平坦无凹凸。清除小路上的青苔与树叶,路潮湿时要特别小心
	51	夜晚时小路与入口处灯光是否明亮	□是	□否	小路与入口处晚上应有明亮的照明
	52	车库的地板是否没有油脂和汽油	□是	□否	车库的地板应没有油脂和汽油
	53	房子周围的公共场所是否修缮良好	□是	□否	公共场所应修缮良好

表 B.11 跌倒风险评估量表

评估项目	评估内容	权重	得分	评估项目	评估内容	权重	得分
活动能力	步态异常/假肢	3		自控能力	失禁	1	
	行走需要辅助设施	3			频率增加	1	
	行走需要旁人帮助	3			保留导尿	1	
精神状态	谵妄	3		跌倒史	有跌倒史	2	
	痴呆	3			因跌倒住院	3	
	兴奋/行为异常	2		用药情况	新药	1	
	神志恍惚	3			心血管药物	1	

表 B.11（续）

评估项目	评估内容	权重	得分	评估项目	评估内容	权重	得分
用药情况	降压药	1			失眠	1	
	镇静、催眠药	1			夜游症	1	
	戒断治疗	1		年龄	年龄 80 岁及以上	3	
	糖尿病药	1			其他	1	
	抗癫痫药	1		相关	神经科疾病	1	
	麻醉药	1		疾病史	骨质疏松症	1	
感觉障碍	视觉受损	1			骨折史	1	
	听觉受损	1			低血压	1	
	感觉性失语	1			药物/酒精戒断	1	
	其他情况	1			缺氧症	1	
睡眠状况	多醒	1			评估总得分		

评定标准：1～2 分为低危；3～9 分为中危；10 分及以上为高危。

表 B.12 Morse 跌倒评估量表

序号	条件	评分	评分细则	得分
1	3 个月内曾有跌倒史/视觉障碍	无＝0 分□ 有＝25 分□	询问患者及照顾者近 3 个月内有无跌倒史，老年患者可能因记忆力下降或怕伤自尊而造成评分不准确	
2	超过一个医疗诊断	无＝0 分□ 有＝15 分□	查询病历记录	
3	使用助行器具	没有需要/完全卧床/需要扶持＝0 分□ 丁形拐杖/手杖/学步车＝15 分□ 扶家具行走＝30 分□	能自己行走，或完全不需要行走 先观察后询问（患者及照顾者）	
4	静脉治疗/置管/使用药物治疗	无＝0 分□ 有＝20 分□	指用麻醉药、抗组胺药、抗高血压药、镇静催眠药、抗癫痫痉挛药、轻泻药、利尿药、降糖药、抗抑郁抗焦虑抗精神病药	
5	步态	正常乏力/卧床/轮椅代步＝0 分□ ≥65 岁/体位性低血压＝10 分□ 失调及不平衡＝20 分□	正常步态或完全卧床患者 双下肢虚弱乏力的患者并不一定出现肌力及功能下降 因神经功能损伤或骨关节疾病等原因造成的一侧或双侧肢体运动感觉功能下降或残疾	
6	精神状态	了解自己的能力＝0 分□ 忘记自己限制/意识障碍/躁动不安/沟通障碍/睡眠障碍＝15 分□	无认知障碍，遵医，可因宣教而改变不良行为 有认知障碍；过于自信，不遵医行为等	

评定标准：＜25 分为低度风险；25～45 分为中度风险；＞45 分为高度风险。

表 B.13　临床痴呆量表（CDR）

内容	健康 CDR＝0	可疑痴呆 CDR＝0.5	轻度痴呆 CDR＝1	中度痴呆 CDR＝2	重度痴呆 CDR＝3
记忆力	无记忆力缺损或只有轻微的、偶尔的健忘	经常性的轻度健忘，对事情能部分回忆，即"良性健忘"	中度记忆缺损，近事遗忘突出，记忆缺损妨碍日常生活	严重记忆缺损，能记住非常熟悉的事情，新发生的事情很快遗忘	严重记忆丧失，仅存片段的记忆
定向力	能完全正确定向	对时间关系有轻微困难，其余能完全正确定向	对时间关系有中度困难，检查时对地点仍有定向力，但在某些场合可能有地理定向能力障碍	对时间关系有严重困难，通常对时间不能定向，常有地点失定向	仅对自身有定向力
判断力解决问题的能力	能很好地解决日常问题，处理事务和财务，判断力良好	在解决问题、辨别事务间的异同点方面有轻微缺损	在解决问题、辨别事务间的异同点方面有中度困难，通常还能维持社交事务判断力	在解决问题、辨别事务间的异同点方面有严重损害，社会判断力通常受损	不能做判断或不能解决问题
社会事务	和往常一样能独立处理工作、购物、参与义务劳动及社会群体活动	在这些活动方面仅有轻微损害	已不能独立进行这些活动，可以从事其中部分活动，不经意地观察似乎正常	没有外出独立活动的愿望　被带到家庭以外的场所仍能参加活动	病重得不能被带到家庭以外的场所参加活动
家庭生活、业余爱好	家庭生活、业余爱好和需要用脑的兴趣均很好保持	家庭生活、业余爱好和需要用脑的兴趣有轻微损害	家庭活动有肯定的轻度障碍，放弃难度大的家务，放弃复杂的爱好和兴趣	仅能做简单家务，兴趣明显受限，而且维持得差	丧失有意义的家庭活动
个人自理能力	完全自理	须旁人督促或提醒	穿衣、个人卫生及个人事务都需要帮助	个人自理方面需要很大帮助，经常大、小便失禁	个人自理方面需要很大帮助，经常大、小便失禁

说明：只有当损害是由于认识缺陷引起时，才记为 0.5、1、2、3。

表 B.14　老年谵妄评估法（CAM）

序号	评估项目	评估方法	评分	得分
1	急性发作且病程波动	1a.与平常相比较，是否有任何证据显示病人精神状态产生急性变化？	否＝0 分 是＝1 分	
		1b.这些不正常的行为是否在一天中呈现波动状态？即症状来来去去或严重程度起起落落	否＝0 分 是＝1 分	
2	注意力不集中	2.病人是否集中注意力有困难？例如容易分心或无法接续刚刚说过的话	否＝0 分 是＝1 分	

表 B.14（续）

序号	评估项目	评估方法	评分	得分
3	思考缺乏组织	3.病人是否思考缺乏组织或不连贯？如杂乱或答非所问的对话、不清楚或不合逻辑的想法、或无预期的从一个主题跳到另一个主题	否＝0分 是＝1分	
4	意识状态改变	4.整体而言,病人的意识状态为过度警觉、嗜睡、木僵或昏迷	否＝0分 是＝1分	

说明:1a、1b、2 皆为"是",且 3 或 4 任何一项为"是",即为谵妄。

表 B.15 微型营养评定法（MNA）

序号	筛查项目	评分方法	得分
1	在过去的 3 个月由于食欲下降、消化系统问题、咀嚼或吞咽困难,使食物摄入减少吗?	0 分＝严重的食物摄入减少 1 分＝中度的食物摄入减少 2 分＝食物摄入无改变	
2	在最近的 3 个月中有体重减轻	0 分＝体重减轻>3 kg 1 分＝不知道 2 分＝体重减轻在 1～3 kg 之间 3 分＝无体重减轻	
3	移动	0 分＝只能在床或椅子上活动 1 分＝能离开床或椅子,但不能外出 2 分＝可以外出	
4	在过去的 3 个月中,遭受心理压力或急性疾病	0 分＝是 2 分＝否	
5	神经心理问题	0 分＝严重的精神紊乱或抑郁 1 分＝中等程度的精神紊乱 2 分＝无神经心理问题	
6	体重指数（BMI）（kg/m^2）	0 分＝BMI<19 1 分＝19≤BMI<21 2 分＝21≤BMI<23 3 分＝BMI≥23	

筛查分数（各分项总分 14 分）:≥12 分,正常-无危险,不需要完成评估;≤11 分,可能有营养不良,继续进行评估

序号	筛查项目	评分方法		
7	生活独立(不住在护理院或医院)	0 分＝否	1 分＝是	
8	每日服用 3 种以上的处方药	0 分＝是	1 分＝否	
9	压伤或皮肤溃疡	0 分＝有	1 分＝否	
10	患者每日进几餐(指一日三餐)	0 分＝1 餐	1 分＝2 餐	2 分＝3 餐

表 B.15（续）

序号	评估项目	评分方法	得分
11	选择摄入蛋白质的消耗量： 每日至少进食牛奶和酸奶中的 1 种(是,否) 每周进食 2 种以上的豆类或蛋类(是,否) 每日进食肉、鱼或禽类(是,否)	0 分＝选择 0 或 1 个是 0.5 分＝选择 2 个是 1 分＝选择 3 个是	
12	每日食用 2 种以上的水果或蔬菜	0 分＝否　　1 分＝是	
13	每日进食液体情况(水、果汁、咖啡、茶、奶等)	0 分＝至少 3 杯 0.5 分＝3～5 杯 1 分＝超过 5 杯	
14	进食的方式	0 分＝必须在帮助下进食 1 分＝独自进食但有些困难 2 分＝独自进食无任何问题	
15	对自己营养状况的认识	0 分＝认为自己有营养不良 1 分＝对自己的营养状况不确定 2 分＝认为自己没有营养问题	
16	患者认为与其他的同龄人相比自己的健康状况如何?	0 分＝不好　　0.5 分＝不知道 1 分＝一样好　2 分＝更好	
17	上臂围 MAC(cm)	0 分＝MAC＜21 0.5 分＝21≤MAC＜22 1 分＝MAC≥22	
18	小腿围 CC(cm)	0 分＝CC＜31　　1 分＝CC≥31	

评估结果_____筛查项目得分_____评估项目得分(最高 16 分)_____总分_____

营养不良指导标准：17～23.5 分,有营养不良的危险；＜17 分,营养不良

表 B.16　营养风险筛查法(NRS2002)

基本情况	姓名		住院号	
	性别		病区	
	年龄		床号	
	身高		体重(kg)	
	体质指数(BMI)		蛋白质(g/L)	
	临床诊断			

	患病种类及病名	分数	得分
疾病状况	骨盆骨折或者慢性病患者合并有以下疾病：肝硬化、慢性阻塞性肺病、长期血液透析、糖尿病肿瘤	1	
	腹部重大手术、中风、重症肺炎、血液系统肿瘤	2	
	颅脑损伤、骨髓抑制、加护病患(APACHE＞10 分)	3	

表 B.16（续）

营养状况指标（单选）		分数	得分
营养状况	正常营养状态	0	
	3 个月内体重减轻＞5％或最近 1 个星期进食量（与需要量相比）减少 20％～50％	1	
	2 个月内体重减轻＞5％或 BMI18.5～20.5 或最近 1 个星期进食量（与需要量相比）减少 50％～75％	2	
	1 个月内体重减轻＞5％（或 3 个月内减轻＞15％）或 BMI＜18.5（或血清白蛋白＜35 g/L）或最近 1 个星期进食量（余需要量相比）减少 70％～100％	3	
年龄	年龄≥70 岁加算 1 分	1	

营养风险筛查总分：_____

评估与干预建议

总分≥3.0,患者有营养不良的风险,需营养支持治疗

总分＜3.0,若患者将接受重大手术,则每周重新评估其营养状况

表 B.17 老年抑郁评估（GDS-5）量表简表

询问被测试者过去一周的情况：

序号	评估内容	评分		得分
1	您对生活基本上满意吗？	是＝0 分	否＝1 分	
2	您是否常常感到厌烦？	是＝1 分	否＝0 分	
3	您是否常常感到无论做什么事都没有用？	是＝1 分	否＝0 分	
4	您是否比较喜欢待在家里,而不喜欢外出和做新的事？	是＝1 分	否＝0 分	
5	您是否觉得您现在活得很没价值？	是＝1 分	否＝0 分	

评估总得分_____

评价标准:2 分以下,正常;≥2 分,可疑有抑郁情形。

表 B.18 老年抑郁评估量表（GDS-15）

询问被测试者过去一周的情况：

序号	评估内容	评分		得分
1	您对您的生活基本上满意吗？	是＝0 分	否＝1 分	
2	您是否常感到厌烦？	是＝1 分	否＝0 分	
3	您是否常常感到无论做什么都没有用？	是＝1 分	否＝0 分	
4	您是否比较喜欢呆在家里而较不喜欢外出及不喜欢做新的事？	是＝1 分	否＝0 分	
5	您是否感到您现在生活的没有价值？	是＝1 分	否＝0 分	
6	您是否减少很多的活动和嗜好？	是＝1 分	否＝0 分	
7	您是否觉得您的生活很空虚？	是＝1 分	否＝0 分	

表 B. 18（续）

序号	评估内容	评分		得分
8	您是否大部分时间精神都很好？	是＝0分	否＝1分	
9	您是否害怕将有不幸的事情发生在您身上？	是＝1分	否＝0分	
10	您是否大部分时间都感到快乐？	是＝0分	否＝1分	
11	您是否觉得您比大多数人有较多记忆的问题？	是＝1分	否＝0分	
12	您是否觉得"现在还能活着"是很好的事情？	是＝0分	否＝1分	
13	您是否觉得精力充沛？	是＝0分	否＝1分	
14	您是否觉得您现在的情况是没有希望？	是＝1分	否＝0分	
15	您是否觉得大部分的人都比您幸福？	是＝1分	否＝0分	
	评估总得分＿＿＿＿＿＿＿			

评价标准：1～4分为不考虑抑郁；5～9分为可能抑郁症；≥10分为抑郁症。

表 B. 19　皮肤危险因子评估表（Braden 量表）

序号	评估项目	评分内容及评分标准				得分
		1 分	2 分	3 分	4 分	
1	意识状况	完全昏迷	昏迷但对痛有反应	清醒但部分感官受损	清醒正常	
2	清洁状况	失禁潮湿	失禁，更换每天≤3 次	失禁，每次更换	干燥、干净	
3	移动能力	完全限制不动	大部分不动	部分限制	没有限制	
4	活动能力	绝对卧床	仅限坐姿（轮椅）	经常下床	自由下床	
5	饮食状况	禁食	摄取量少于 1 200 cal/d	摄取量可达需要量的一半以上，管饲或全胃肠外营养（TPN）能达到绝大部分营养所需	摄取量≥需要量	
6	摩擦力和剪切力	有问题	有潜在问题	没问题		
	评估总得分（分值范围 6～23 分）＿＿＿＿＿＿＿					

评价标准：15～18 分为低危；13～14 分为中危；10～12 分为高危；≤9 分为极高危。

参 考 文 献

[1] 中华人民共和国民政部.老年人能力评估标准:MZ/T 039—2013[S/OL].北京:中国标准出版社

[2] 护理院基本标准,卫医政发〔2011〕21号

[3] 中国康复辅助器具目录,2014年6月4日

[4] 全国医院信息化建设标准与规范(试行),国家卫生健康委员会规划与信息司与国家卫生健康委员会统计信息中心,2018年4月

[5] 宋惠平,陈峥.老年友善医院[J].中华老年医学杂志.2016,8(35):1018-21

[6] 宋岳涛,陈峥,高茂龙,等.北京市老年友善医院标准解读[J].中国老年保健医学杂志,2018,16(3):11-15

[7] 周燕珉等.养老设施建筑设计详解[M].中国建筑工业出版社,2018

[8] 宋岳涛,金哲,高茂龙等.医疗服务机构老年综合评估基本标准与服务规范(试行)[J].中国老年保健医学杂志,2018,16(3):3-10

[9] 宋岳涛.老年综合评估(第二版)[M],北京:中国协和医科大学出版社,2019

[10] World Health Organization. Global Age-friendly Cities:A Guide. Publication date:2007. ISBN:978 92 4 154730 7. http://www.who.int/kobe_centre/publications/age_friendly_cities_guide/en/

[11] World Health Organization. WHO age-friendly environments,programme. http://www.who.int/ageing/age_friendly_cities/en/index.html

[12] World Health Organization. Age-friendly Primary Health Care Centres Toolkit. http://www.who.int/ageing/publications/Age-Friendly-PHC-Centre-toolkitDec08.pdf

[13] World Health Organization. Active Aging:Towards Age-friendly Primary Health Care. http://www.who.int/hpr/ageing

[14] Health Promotion Administration,Ministry of Health and Welfare:Age-friendly Hospitals and Health Services Recognition Self-assessment. Manual http://www.hpa.gov.tw/BHPNet/Web/HealthTopic/TopicArticle.aspx

[15] Regional Geriatric Program of Toronto,Senior Friendly Hospitals,A Toolkit for Senior Friendly Hospitals. RGP;2011. http://senior friendly hospitals.ca

ICS 03.080
A 20

Social Organization Standard

T/CGSS 003—2019

Specification for age-friendly service

老年友善服务规范

（*English Translation*）

Issue date：2019-03-01   Implementation date：2019-03-01

Issued by   Chinese Geriatrics Society

Foreword

This standard was drafted in accordance with the rules given in GB/T 1.1—2009.

This standard was proposed by Beijing Geriatric Hospital.

This standard was prepared by Chinese Geriatrics Society.

This standard was drafted by Beijing Geriatric Hospital，Geriatric Medical Institution Management Branch of China Geriatrics Society，Beijing Medical Association's Geriatrics Training and Counseling Center，Liaoning Province Geriatric Hospital(Liaoning Province Jinqiu Hospital)，Geriatric Hospital of Zhengzhou（Ninth People's Hospital of Zhengzhou ），Jiangsu Province Geriatric Hospital，Hebei Province Geriatric Hospital，Hainan Province Geriatric Hospital，Chengdu Eighth People's Hospital，Chengdu Elderly Care Hospital，Sichuan Zigong Fifth People's Hospital，Leshan Geriatrics Specialist Hospital，Yunnan Rehabilitation Hospital（Kunming Geriatric Hospital），Sinopharm Dongfeng Huaguo Hospital，Inner Mongolia Kerqin District Geriatric Hospital，Zibo Zijian Group Hospital，Daqing Oilfield Donghai Hospital，Tangshan Workers Group Hospital，Taiyuan Municipal No.2 Peoples Hospital and Beijing Dongcheng District Integrative Medicine Hospital.

The main drafters of this standard were Yuetao Song，Zheng Chen，Jinping Zhang，Shuangqiu Liu，Huiping Song，Baoying Li，Jimin Bao，Jianlin Bai ，Jiaren Xu，Jianjun Liu，Shuijing Jin，Weihong Bi，Daizhi Peng，Hongsong Xiao ，Youguo Tan，Bin Zhu，Fujian Tian，Wanbao Hu ，Xiaohong Mu，Xiaoyun Deng ，Chunlin Zhang ，Yujie Li and Yanli Lu.

Specification for age-friendly service

1 Scope

This standard specifies basic requirements, services and requirements, service evaluation and improvement of age-friendly service.

This standard is applicable to medical and rehabilitation institutes, nursing homes and other care service providers.

2 Normative references

The following referenced documents are indispensable for the application of this document. For dated references, only the edition cited applies. For undated references, the latest edition of the referenced document (including any amendments) applies.

GB/T 16432 Assistive products for persons with disability—Classification and terminology.

GB/T 17242 Guidelines for complaints handling.

T/CGSS 001 Specification for elderly caregiver.

3 Terms and definitions

. For the purposes of this document, the terms and definitions given in GB/T 16432 and the following apply.

3.1
age-friendly service

activities and services provided by medical and rehabilitation institutes, nursing home and other care service providers that are designed to meet special needs for the elderly in a respectful, caring and supportive environment.

3. 2
comprehensive geriatric assessment

a multidisciplinary assessment process that requires evaluation of multiple issues, including physical, cognitive, psychological, social, environmental and disease components that influence the health of an elderly with physical impairments and decreased muscle strength.

3. 3
inter-disciplinary integrated management

a comprehensive model of medical, rehabilitation and care service that is implemented for elderly patients by a multidisciplinary medical team consisting of geriatricians, rehabilitation physicians and therapists, nurses, psychologists, dietitians, clinical pharmacists, case managers and social workers based on the results of the comprehensive assessment of the elderly.

3. 4
geriatric syndrome
GS

an aging condition with common clinical manifestations caused by a variety of chronic pathological aging or multiple predisposing factors.

4 Basic requirements

4. 1 Service provider organizations

4. 1. 1 Service provider organizations ("providers") include hospitals, rehabilitation centers, nursing homes, pension agencies, and nursing care centers that provide multiple medical services, etc.

4. 1. 2 Legal registration is required.

4. 1. 3 Providers shall have management departments and staff who are designated to serve the elderly, and maintain care-providing systems, procedures, service specifications and emergency plans.

4. 1. 4 It is required to establish a reporting and feedback system to manage information of adverse events in age-friendly services according to the *National Hospital Informationization Construction Standards and Specifications* (*Trial*).

4. 1. 5 A designated management department with full-time staff is required to be responsible for the two-way referral services.

4. 1. 6 The service personnel shall be trained on safety knowledge and skills training before and during employment, and are required to take no less than 20 hours of training per year. All training assessment shall meet the requirements prior to the employment.

4.1.7 It is recommended to operate independently or cooperatively a long-term care ward or elderly care home for the elderly. The operation guidance should be in accordance with *Basic Standards for Nursing Homes*.

4.1.8 It is recommended to establish organizations and management systems such as social work department and volunteer department. Ther is a long-term plan for recruiting volunteers, especially elderly volunteers.

4.1.9 The original medical records and related documents shall be preserved properly and confidentially for record tracking.

4.2 Service personnel

4.2.1 All personnel shall provide health certificates, conduct professional ethics, respect the ethnic customs and religious beliefs of the elderly, and protect personal privacy and information security of the elderly.

4.2.2 All personnel shall have the ability to communicate effectively with the elderly. To communicate with the elderly with physical and mental disabilities, it is recommended to speak slowly and clearly and use body languages, images or letters. Volunteers, patients and their families are supported and encouraged to participate in inter-disciplinary integrated management of the elderly healthcare.

4.2.3 Technical personnel shall have relevant qualifications, participate in relevant training, and understand safety conduct in technical operations and hygiene requirements of the facilities.

4.2.4 Medical personnel shall have diagnostic skills and provide treatments for common senile diseases, conduct comprehensive assessment for the elderly, provide risk screening and intervention plans for the geriatric syndromes, and provide free consultation, disease screening, and health education activities for the elderly on a regular basis.

4.2.5 Nursing staff shall have comprehensive assessment skills for the elderly, develop personalized nursing plans based on the evaluation results, and provide the elderly or their guardians judgment and recommenda-tions for treatments and elderly care management plans appropriate for home, community , nursing home,or admission treatment.

4.2.6 The director level personnel of the Department of Geriatrics and related specialties shall be at least the associate chief physician level with an educational background in geriatrics or physicians meeting the training requirements in geriatric practice. The supervisor of nursing personnel shall hold the title of senior supervisor or above in the elderly nursing practice.

4.2.7 Rehabilitation therapists shall hold intermediate-level or above professional certificates in related fields. The supervision-level personnel shall hold at least the intermediate level of professional and technical titles ,and are required to have practice experience of 5 years or more.

4.2.8 The elderly medication and nutrition consultation shall be provided through outpatient visits by medical professionals with 5 years or more of relevant clinical experience.

4.2.9 All elderly caregivers shall follow the guidance provided in T/CGSS 001.

4.3 Environment and facilities

4.3.1 Environment providing age-friendly services shall be safe and convenient with facilities such as mobility aids and accessible bathrooms to meet the needs of their older residents with physical impairments and congnitive disabilities by considering their physiological, pathophysiological and functional factors.

4.3.2 Mobility aids shall be available for public use within the facility, the service information shall be placed in a prominent location and be easy for the elderly to read and understand.

4.3.3 The general environment of the facility, the indoor environment of medical wards, bathrooms, hallways and elevators environment,transportation facilities and sign systems should meet the age-friendly criteria for service providers. See details in annex A,table A.1.

5 Services and requirements

5.1 Comprehensive geriatric assessment

5.1.1 The institute shall conduct the comprehensive geriatric assessment and evaluation for the elderly. The evaluation contents and methods are shown in Table 1.

5.1.2 A medical intervention plan shall be provided by assessors based on the assessment results, and if necessary, the intervention plans may involve joint effort from multidisciplinary medical teams.

5.1.3 It is recommended to evaluate the safety of living environment and provide suggestions for home improvement for elderly patients who are discharged from the hospital. Home safety evaluation shall include assessments of lighting, floor, bathroom, kitchen, living room, bedroom, corridor and hallways. The Family Risk Factor Assessment Tool（HFHA）,see annex B,table B.10.

5.1.4 The assessment results shall be included in the medical records or service files, and the data shall be properly stored and aggregated for analysis.

Table 1 Contents and methods of the comprehensive geriatric assessment

Number	Evaluation content	Evaluation form or tool
1	General medical assessment	Including assessment of illness and medication, see table B. 1
2	Assessment of daily physical activities	Basic daily living activity assessment scale (Barthel Index), see table B. 2
3	Balance function assessment	Balance test, see table B.3 Forearm extension test,see table B. 4
4	Cognitive function assessment	Mini cognitive scale (Mini-Cog), see table B. 5 Mini-mental state examination (MMSE), see table B. 6
5	Vision assessment	Simple vision assessment, see table B. 7
6	Hearing assessment	Simple hearing assessment , see table B. 8
7	Social adaptability assessment	Simple assessment method of social engagement (see the Ministry of Civil Affairs *Evaluation Standards for Senior Citizens*),see table B. 9
8	Home safety assessment	Family risk factor assessment tool (HFHA), see table B. 10

5.2 Evaluation and interventions of geriatric syndromes and elderly care practice

5.2.1 Geriatric syndromes include falls, dementia, delirium, weakness, sarcopenia, polypharmacy, depression, syncope, urinary incontinence, Parkinson's syndromes, constipation, sleep disorders, and chronic pain, etc. Elderly care providers often handle conditions like deep venous thrombosis, pulmonary embolism, pressure ulcers, osteoporosis and fractures, and aspiration pneumonia, etc.

5.2.2 Caregivers shall evaluate and assess geriatric syndromes and conditions. Common assessment of geriatric syndromes and elderly care conditions are shown in Table 2.

5.2.3 The institution shall propose and implement targeted intervention measures based on the assessment results of geriatric syndrome and elderly care issues, such as developing and implementing prevention and control measures for elderly fall risk or treatment measures for fall injury, developing and implementing interventions for prevention and treatment of Alzheimer's disease, senile delirium and geriatric depression, providing prescriptions of nutrition and exercise for malnutrition conditions, preventing and controlling the risk of pressure ulcers for elderly patients with conditions limiting their ability to change positions or implementing correct and effective treatment and care for the long term bedridden elderly patients who have developed pressure ulcers.

5.2.4 The intervention measures for the elderly syndrome and nursing problems should be evaluated effectively.

Table 2 Common assessment of geriatric syndromes and elderly care issues

Number	Evaluation content	Evaluation form
1	Fall risk assessment	Fall risk assessment scale, see table B. 11
		Morse fall assessment scale, see table B. 12
2	Dementia assessment	Mini-mental state examination（MMSE）, see table B. 6
		Clinical dementia rating（CDR）, see table B. 13
3	Delirium assessment	Confusion assessment method（CAM）, see table B. 14
4	Malnutrition assessment	Mini nutritional assessment（MNA）, see table B. 15
		Nutritional risk screening 2002（NRS2002）, see table B. 16
5	Depression assessment	Geriatric depression scale-5（GDS-5）, see table B. 17
		Geriatric depression scale-15（GDS-15）,see table B. 18
6	Pressure ulcer assessment	Braden scale, see table B. 19

5.3 Detection of high-risk state and treatment

5.3.1 Monitoring and identification shall be conducted for high-risk indicators such as falls, falling out of bed, asphyxia, and pulmonary embolism of the elderly. In addition to informing patients, family members and caregivers of the risks, risk identification and other corresponding preventive measures shall also be taken.

5.3.2 Care givers shall have emergency rescue measures for acute stroke, acute myocardial infarction, hypertensive crisis, heart failure, respiratory failure, and renal failure.

5.4 Prevention and control of common diseases in the elderly

5.4.1 Caregivers shall have the prevention and control measures for common diseases in the elderly including but not limited to hypertension, diabetes, hyperlipidemia, stroke, coronary heart disease, chronic obstructive pulmonary disease, pulmonary infection, joint disease, advanced tumor, and chronic kidney disease.

5.4.2 Comprehensive prevention and control of chronic diseases in the elderly shall be implemented, and interventions including exercise and diet plans shall be adopted for high-risk groups. Intervention events shall be documented, along with event notifications, topics, sponsors, audience and live videos or photos, etc.

5.4.3 It is recommended to organize health science education base of common geriatric diseases. Designated personnel including both full-time and part-time staff are responsible for making activity plans, organizing events and recording. Care provider facilities should be equipped with functional devices and materials of health education.

5.5 Medication evaluation for the elderly

5.5.1 Caregivers shall perform comprehensive assessments of medication uses for the elderly（see table B. 1）and provide guidance to prevent any unreasonable medication.

5.5.2 Precautions for all medication shall be provided to the elderly patients who leave the institution.

5.6 Inter-disciplinary integrated management

5.6.1 It is recommended to provide inter-disciplinary integrated management service for the elderly patients with complex conditions，multi-medication uses，multi-system dysfunctions，and multi-organ failures.

5.6.2 Discussions from multidisciplinary medical group meetings shall be documented in order to provide an integrated health management and complication prevention plan for the elderly.

5.6.3 Medical staff and caregivers shall encourage the elderly patients and their families to participate in multidisciplinary group meetings and related activities.

5.7 Geriatric specialist services

5.7.1 Medical care and rehabilitation services should be provided for the elderly patients with Guillain-Barré syndrome（GBS），stroke，cognitive impairment，osteoarthritis，falls，sleep disorders，pressure ulcers，mental disorders，etc.

5.7.2 Nutrition intervention services should be provided for the elderly. Relevant education and prescription of nutrition should be provided based on nutritional risk assessment results.

5.7.3 The elderly patients should be provided with intermediate care，long-term care，hospice care，and other services.

5.7.4 It is recommended to provide the assessment of living conditions and living products and aids for the elderly. Please see *China Rehabilitation Aids Catalogue* for configuration.

5.7.5 Medical records and service records shall be documented for specialized geriatric services.

5.8 Extended services

5.8.1 Extended services refer to continuous medical，nursing，functional rehabilitation and social support services for the elderly returning home or back to their communities after being discharged from hospital. The main service contents and requirements are shown in Table 3.

5.8.2 Extended services shall have service records and effect evaluation.

Table 3 The main service contents and requirements

Number	Service Content	Extended service requirements
1	Continuous care plan	It shall include at least health education, rehabilitation training for daily living activities, dietary guidance, exercise intervention, management of hypertension, diabetes and other chronic diseases
2	Two-way referral service	The management department and full-time personnel responsible for two-way referral services shall provide the elderly patients with referral services after assessment
3	Follow-up service	The hospital outpatient service shall be provided for the elderly patients or network outpatient service should be provided to make appointments for follow-up consultations
4	Green channel	Green channels (expediate services) shall be provided for the elderly under special circumstances for registration, payment, waiting, prescription and examination
5	Health management	Health records and service records shall be documented for providers such as in-home contracted care, pension institutions or other long-term care institutions
6	Technical support	On-site technical support or telemedicine services shall be provided to the medical staff of health service institutions or pension institutions in nearby communities

6 Service evaluation and improvement

6.1 Service evaluation

6.1.1 The evaluation includes Clause 4 and Clause 5 of this standard.

6.1.2 Service evaluation includes care giver self-evaluation, customer evaluation, and third-party evaluation.

—Care giver self-evaluation shall be conducted regularly based on the service contents and service requirements.

—Care giver organization shall regularly evaluate the customers' satisfaction.

—Chinese Geriatrics Society may entrust qualified third-party institutions to conduct evaluations of age-friendly services.

6.2 Improvement

6.2.1 Based on the evaluation results, the organization shall modify executive plans for programs that do not meet the requirements, keep track of the implementation progress, improve continuously service quality in a timely manner.

6.2.2 The organization shall collect information and feedback of service quality issues at any time, analyze the root cause, apply corrections, and modify the process and management to avoid recurrence of mistakes.

6.2.3 The organization shall accept actively social supervision, make the supervision and complaint telephone number available to the public, publish procedures of filing complaints, establish dispute and complaints handling processes, and give feedback solicitation according to the requirements of GB/T 17242.

Annex A

(Informative)

Age-friendly service environment and facilities

Age-friendly service environment and facilities see Table A. 1.

Table A. 1 Age-friendly service environment and facilities

Number	project	Age-friendly service environment and facilities
1	Overall environment	The overall environment needs to remain clean, comfortable and safe
		Floor, wall, furniture with appropriately warm color. Doors, armrest should be distinguished by high contrast color. Floor material should be non-reflective and slip-resistant. Exaggerated geometrical design such as stripesof floor pattern is not recommended
		All wards shall be quiet and be equipped with ventilation system
		Automatic damper delay of the electric door is more than 4 seconds
2	Ward environment	Lighting of the wards should be balanced and sufficient without rotation Night-lights are required
		Window restrictors should be installed in all wards and public areas
		The distance between ward beds should ensure a minimum turn-around space of a wheelchair. The height of the bed should be 100%~120% of the patient's calf length (allowing feet firmly touching on the floor whiling sitting in bed). The bed rails should be approximately 350 mm taller than the mattress. Pressure-relief mattresses and seat cushions should be prepared for long-term bedridden patients
		A bedside pager is installed and buttons are easily accessible. Bed light switch should be obvious and easy to use
		Time and date in a large font size should be presented in silent devices or monitors installed in the wards. High-risk patients should be identifiable
3	Toilet and bathroom environment	Accessible toilet stalls are required for each bathroom (a minimum of 1~2 stalls is required for each ward). Barrier-free and gender-neutral toilets should be accessible in public areas such as outpatient clinics
		Fixed or upturned safety rails should be installed on the front side of the toilet, the recommended horizontal distance between the safety rails and the centerline of the toilet is 350 mm ~ 400 mm, and when lowered down, the upturned safety rails should be 700 mm above the ground. The L-shaped safety rails should be installed on the side walls of the toilet. The centerline of the toilet is 450 mm away from the wall; the vertical segment of the L-shaped rail is 200 mm ~ 250 mm away from the front edge of the toilet; the highest point is more than 1 400 mm away from the ground; and the horizontal segment is 700 mm away from the ground

Table A. 1 (*continued*)

Number	project	Age-friendly service environment and facilities
3	Toilet and bathroom environment	Infusion pump stand should be installed on both sides of the toilet. It is advisable to install call button or pull cord emergency call device on the side wall, the call button is 400 mm ~ 500 mm above ground, and the end of the pull cord is 100mm away from the ground for easy access. A designated person should be responsible for emergency response at any time
		Bathroom doors should have a width ≥900 mm and should be two-way or push open doors. Washbasin should be no lower than 650 mm. All bathrooms should be wheelchair accessible
		Public bathrooms should be equipped with facilities available for patients with or without self-bathing abilities. The wheelchair accessable bathrooms should have enough space for turning around wheelchairs. Toilet or toilet seat should be installed in shower areas. Slip-resistant shower mats should be used in the shower. The height of the shower/shower switch should be convenient for wheelchair users
		Upturned or L-shaped safety rails shall be installed on the sides of toilets, urinals, showers, and bathtubs at a proper position
4	Furniture, handrails, passageways, and elevators environment	Caster brake wheels shall be installed for bedside furniture. Protection cushions should be installed on the sharp edges of the furniture. Dining tables should be adjustable for wheelchairs. All chairs should be slip-resistant, easy to clean and height-adjustable with armrests and soft cushions
		Safety handrails are required on both sides of stairs and corridors. At least one side of ramps should have handrails. A safety sign is required within 100 mm at the end of the ramp
		The appropriate ratio of ramp height to length should be 1:20. A rest platform should be built when the ramp length is over 9m
		A lounge area or chairs are required in a hallway with a length of more than 50 m and any corner of a stairway
		The width of the walkway and ramp should be able to allow two wheelchairs to pass through side by side, and there should be no height difference on the ground, so that wheelchairs and crutches can avoid being gotten stuck
		There shall be clearly identifiable signs on the floor at the beginning and the end of ramps and stairs
		The elevator emergency call buttons should be in bright color and with large font. switch Damping delay of levator door is more than 4 seconds. Safety handrails should be installed on three sides of the elevator walls

Table A. 1 (*continued*)

Number	project	Age-friendly service environment and facilities
5	Traffic facilities	The main entrance and exit of the hospital, outpatient clinic and ward area should be equipped with a barrier-free passageway, and there should be a reserved area for temporary parking for the elderly to get on and off the vehicle
		Safety signs should be found at stairs, ramps and hallway corners, such as speed limit, no honking, sharp turn and deceleration
		Transportation equipment (such as wheelchair, stretcher bed, etc.) should be available for patients to use in outpatient and emergency room and inpatient wards
6	Sign system	Guide signs with great color contrast should be set at the main road crossing, the main entrance and exit of the building and each floor of the courtyard. The colors, fonts, and materials should be consistently used for all signs. Current location shall be provided on the guide signs as well
		Signs should be in plain language with simple graphics. The font size of small sign shall be at least 40 mm ,and the font size of large sign shall be 60 mm
		There shall be clearly identifiable signs on the floor at the beginning and the end of ramps and stairs

Annex B

(informative)

Geriatric comprehensive assessment scale

Geriatric comprehensive assessment scale are shown Table B. 1~Table B. 19.

Table B. 1   General medical assessment

Number	Evaluation content	Evaluation results		
1	Disease evaluation	1. 4. 7. 10.	2. 5. 8. 11.	3. 6. 9. 12.
2	Medication evaluation	1. 4. 7. 10.	2. 5. 8. 11.	3. 6. 9. 12.

Table B. 2   Assessment of activities of daily living (Barthel Index)

Number	Items	Explanation	Scales	Goal
1	Fecal incontinence (fecal)	Refers to the condition within 1 week occasionally = once a week	0 = no control of bowels 5 = occasional loss of control (<1 time per week), or need help from others 10 = be able to control and have no accidents	
2	Urinary incontinence (urinary)	Refers to condition within 24 h~48 h "Occasionally" refers to <1 time/day	0 = completely out of control, or with an indwelling catheter urination control 5 = occasionally out of control (<1 time per day, more than once per week), or need help from others 10 = be able to control and have no accidents, or patients with catheter can complete independently the release and closure of the catheter	
3	Grooming (refers to wash face, brush teeth, comb hair, and shave , etc.)	Refers to condition within 24 h~48 h	0 = need help from others 5 = be able to complete activities independently, or with the tools being provided by the caregiver, such as squeezing toothpaste, preparing water, etc	

Table B. 2 （*continued*）

Number	Items	Explanation	Scales	Goal
4	Toilet use （including walk to the toilet, handling clothes, wipe, flush）	The patient shall be able to complete the whole process of going to the toilet independently	0 = need great help or total dependent on others 5 = need some help （need someone's help to walk to the bathroom, or need someone to help flush or organize clothes, etc. ） 10 = be able to complete activities independently	
5	Feeding （refers to the process of transfer food from the container to the mouth, chew, swallow, etc. ）	The patient shall be able to complete the whole process of eating independently, food can be prepared or served by other people	0 = needs great help or total dependence on others, or has a feeding tube 5 = need some help （needs some help, such as cutting up the food, preparing utensil and serving dishes to table, etc. ） 10 = can finish eating independently （within a reasonable time to finish eating independently）	
6	Transfers （walking between bed and chair）	Walking from bed to chair and back, including sitting in bed	0 = totally dependent on others, unable to sit 5 = need great help （2 people）, be able to sit （with a higher degree of dependence on others ） 10 = need some help （1 person） or support （need someone to help or use crutches） 15 = can move independently	
7	Walking on the ground （walking）	Refers to activities within hospital or indoor with the help of auxiliary tools. If you use a wheelchair, you must be able to turn around or travel on your own without assistance	0 = rely on others completely 5 = need great help （ rely on others in a great degree for help due to physical disability, poor balance, excessive weakness, poor vision, etc. or moving in a wheelchair） 10 = need some help （ need help from others to some extent due to physical disability, poor balance, excessive weakness, poor vision, etc. , or use crutches, walking aids and other auxiliary equipment） 15 = can walk 45 minutes independently on the level surface	
8	Dressing（refers to putting on and taking off clothes, shoes and sock, fastening, zipping, and tying shoes,etc. ）	Be able to dress himself up independently	0 = need great help or total dependence on others 5 = need some help （be able to put on and take off independently, but need others to help dress up） 10 = can be complete activities independently （buttoning, zippering, taking off-shoes, etc. ）	
9	Climbing stairs		0 = can't be able to climb stairs 5 = need some help （physical or verbal guidance） 10 = be able to complete activities independently	

Table B. 2 (*continued*)

Number	Items	Explanation	Scales	Goal
10	Bathing	Be able to turn on water faucet, adjust water temperature, apply bath and rinse and other bathing actions independently	0 = rely on other's help 5 = be able to complete activities independently	
Total evaluation score:				

Evaluation criteria: 100 points: complete independency; 65~95 points: mild dependency; 45~60 points: moderate dependency; ≤ 40 points: severe dependency.

Description: The total score is 100 points. The result shows the higher the score, the higher degree of independency a patient has.

Table B. 3 Balance Test

Number	Test method	Evaluation method	Time of standing
1	Feet together stand	Stand with two feet together side by side	seconds
2	Semi-tandem stand	Stand with two feet together side by side with one foot placed in front with half foot distance from the other	seconds
3	Tandem stand	Stand with two feet in a straight line, the heel of the front foot is close to the toe of the other one	seconds

Evaluation criteria: Time of Tandem standing is less than 10 seconds, suggesting poor balance function and risk of falling.

Table B. 4 Forearm extension test

Test method	Thresholds	Functional evaluation
1. The patient should stand still and upstraight against the wall, then lift up both arms up to 90 degree angle with palms facing down and close both hands to fists. Patient should try to extend both fists forward as much as possible. 2. Measure the distance between third metacarpal bone and the wall three times, and take the average value as the final result. Make sure to prevent the patient from falling during the evaluation.	≤12 cm	Very poor balance function, high risk of falling
	<15 cm	Poor balance and risk of falling
	20~25 cm	Balance function is somewhat good
	≥25 cm	Good balance function
Description: The normal reference value shall be ≥15 cm.		

Table B. 5 Mini cognitive scale（Mini-Cog）

Items	Test content and results	Grading	Score
Instructions	A. "I have three things：apple、watch and flag. I want you to repeat back to me now and try to remember. I'll ask you later.."	—	—
	B. Clock drawing："Please draw a clock and set the hands to 10 past 11."		
	C. Three work recall："Please tell me what the three things I asked you to remember were?"		
Answers	Answer：___，___，___ （need not in order）	—	—
Result interpretation	Draw the clock correctly（draw a closed circle、the positions of hands are accurate）、and can recall 3 words	3	
	Draw the clock correctly（draw a closed circle、the positions of hands are accurate）、and can recall 1～2 words	2	
	Draw the clock inaccurately（the circle is not closed、or the positions of hands are not accurate）、or only 1～2 words are recalled	1	
	If a patient cannot recall any word、a diagnosis of cognitive impairment such as dementia is suggested	0	
Evaluation criteria：2 points and above、no dementia；1 point、potential dementia；0 point：dementia.			

Table B.6 Mini-mental state examination(MMSE)

Test item	Number	Evaluation items	Evaluation method	Score
Time	1	What is the year now?	1 for correct、0 for wrong or rejected	
	2	what is the season now?	same as above	
	3	What is the month now?	same as above	
	4	what is the date today?	same as above	
	5	What day is it today?	same as above	
Location	6	What city is this?	same as above	
	7	What is this district?	same as above	
	8	What is this hospital(name of hospital or alley)?	same as above	
	9	What floor is this?	same as above	
	10	What is this place (address、room number)?	same as above	

Table B. 6 （continued）

Test item	Number	Evaluation items	Evaluation method	Score
Memory	\multicolumn{4}{l}{Instructions: Now I will tell you the names of three things. Please repeat after me and remember them: ball, flag and tree, I will ask you later （ Give a full second for each item）}	
	11	Repeat:ball	1 for correct, 0 for wrong or rejected	
	12	Repeat:flag	same as above	
	13	Repeat:tree	same as above	
Attention and calculation	\multicolumn{4}{l}{Instructions: Now please do the continuous calculation of 100 minus 7. Please tell me the answer after each minus 7 until I say "stop"}	
	14	Calculate 100-7 = ?	1 for correct, 0 for wrong	
	15	Calculate again	1 for correct, 0 for wrong	
	16	Calculate again	1 for correct, 0 for wrong	
	17	Calculate again	1 for correct, 0 for wrong	
	18	Calculate again	1 for correct, 0 for wrong	
	\multicolumn{4}{l}{Notes: If the previous item is calculated incorrectly, but the result is correct based on the incorrect caculation , the corresponding score is still given}	
Recall	\multicolumn{4}{l}{Instruction: Now, please tell me the three things I just asked you to remember?}	
	19	Recall:ball	. 1 for correct, 0 for wrong or rejected	
	20	Recall:flag	. same as above	
	21	Recall:tree	. same as above	
	22	The examiner presents a watch to ask the patient what it is	same as above	
	23	The examiner presents a pencil and asks the patient what it is	same as above	
	24	Please speak after me "Can you can a can as a canner can a can"	1 for correctly speaking, 0 for otherwise	
	25	The examiner gives the patient a card with the words as "Please close your eyes. " Please ask the patient to read this sentence and do what it says	1 for correctly speaking and acting,0 for otherwise	

Table B. 6（*continued*）

Test item	Number	Evaluation items	Evaluation method	Score
Language skills		Instruction: I will give you a piece of paper and please follow my instructions. Starting now, hold the paper with your right hand and fold the paper in half with two hands, then place it on your left leg		
	26	Hold this paper with the right hand	1 for correct action, 0 for wrong	
	27	Fold the paper in half with two hands	1 for correct action, 0 for wrong	
	28	Put the paper on your left leg	1 for correct action, 0 for wrong	
	29	Please write a complete sentence.	1 for correct action, 0 for wrong	
	30	Please copy this picture. 	1 for correct action, 0 for wrong	
Total evaluation score:				
Description: The total score ranges from 0 to 30 points. The normal and abnormal cut-off scores are related to the level of education: 17 points for the illiterate (uneducated) group;20 points for patients with primary school education (years of education ≤ 6);24 points for patients with secondary education or above (years of education > 6). Patients who are scored less than the cut-off scores are considered with potential cognitive disorderswhereas patients who are scored above the cut-off scores are considered to be normal.				

Table B. 7　Simple vision assessment

Number	Evaluation items	Grading	Score
1	Be able to see the standard font on books and newspapers	4	
2	Can read large font clearly,but can not read the standard font on books and newspapers	3	
3	With vision limitation and not be able to see newspapers' headlines, but be able to identify general objects	2	
4	With difficulty in identifying an object, but be able to follow a moving object and sensible to light, color and shape.	1	
5	No vision and notb e able to follow any moving object	0	
Total evaluation score:			
Description: Patients swearing prescription glasses or presbyopic glasses for daily activities should be tested with glasses. Recommended evaluation criteria: 4: normal vision; 3: low vision; 1~2: blind; 0: completely blind.			

Table B. 8　Simple hearing assessment

Number	Evaluation items	Grading	Score
1	Be able to communicate well, and hear the sound of TV, telephone, and doorbell	4	
2	Be unable to hear clearly if speaking softly or at a distance of more than 2 meters	3	
3	Be unable to communicate in a normal way and only be able to hear if speaking in a quiet environment or speaking loudly	2	
4	Be able to hear partially if speaking loudly and slowly	1	
5	Completely deaf	0	

Description:Patients wearing hearing aids should be tested with hearing aids.
Recommended evaluation criteria: 4: normal hearing; 3: hearing loss; 1~2: hearing impairment; 0: complete deafness.

Table B. 9　Simple assessment of social engagement

Number	Evaluation items	Grading	Score
1	Participate in social activities, have certain adaptability to social environment, and treat people appropriately	4	
2	Be able to adapt to a simple social environment, be able to actively engage with people. It is difficult for people to find out the intelligence problems when they first meet.. Be unable to understand metaphoric meaning of a language	3	
3	Be unable to adapt to any social environment,be unable to engage actively with people but be able to engage passively with people, inappropriate use of language in communication and easy to be deceived	2	
4	Be barely able to communicate with people, be unable to deliver clear messages in communication and properly manage facial expression	1	
5	Be unable to engage with people	0	

Evaluation criteria: 4: full engagement; 3:slightly reduced engagement ; 2: moderately reduced engagement; 0~1: loss of social engagement.

Table B. 10　Family risk factor assessment tool（HFHA）and recommendations

Items	Number	Evaluation items	Result	Recommendation
Indoor lighting	1	Is the room lighting suitable	☐Yes ☐No	The lighting should not be too bright or too dark
	2	Are the lights of the corridors and stairs bright enough	☐Yes ☐No	To use a 60-watt bulb for passage ways and stair cases. Lights with photoelectric control should be installed for the passage ways

Table B. 10 (*continued*)

Items	Number	Evaluation items	Result	Recommendation
Indoor lighting	3	Is the light switch easy to reach	☐Yes ☐No	The light should be easily switched on and off
	4	Is it easy to reach the light switch from bed	☐Yes ☐No	It should be easy to reach the light switch from bed
	5	Is the storage place with enough lighting	☐Yes ☐No	Lights should be installed for dark areas. Intentionally slow transition from dark to bright area is recommended
Ground (floor)	6	Is the ground level	☐Yes ☐No	The ground should be level, otherwise, it should be smoothed by using a ramp or a slope. Tall door sills are not recommended
	7	Is the carpet (mat) flat, without wrinkles and curling at the edges	☐Yes ☐No	Make sure the carpet (mat) is in good condition and discard the worn or curled carpet
	8	Is the floor slippery and hard	☐Yes ☐No	The floor (board) should not be slippery, it can be applied with slip-resistant agent, and carpeted
	9	Does the floor mat slip	☐Yes ☐No	Remove any loose floor mats or secure them to the floor and apply a non-slip mat pad
	10	Do you wipe away any spilled liquid immediately	☐Yes ☐No	Wipe and clean up any spilled liquid immediately
	11	Is there something messy on the floor	☐Yes ☐No	The floor should be clean with no trip, and fall risks corridors should not be blocked by any obstacles
	12	Are there any wires in the passageway	☐Yes ☐No	There should be no wires in the passageway
Bathroom	13	Is the slip-resistant mat used in the bathtub or bathroom	☐Yes ☐No	Wet floor can be slippery. Anti-slip mats should be used in the bathroom, and non-slip material should be used in the bathtub
	14	Are toiletries easy to reach	☐Yes ☐No	All toiletries should be placed in the area that is easy to reach
	15	Are handrails installed for toilet, bathtub and shower	☐Yes ☐No	Proper handrails should be provided
	16	Is it easy to sit down on the toilet and stand up	☐Yes ☐No	The toilet should not be too low for the elderly to sit on. A toilet booster and proper armrests are recommended for install
	17	Is the bathtub too high	☐Yes ☐No	The bathtub should not be too high. If it is too high, you should add a bath stool or a bath chair

Table B. 10 (*continued*)

Items	Number	Evaluation items	Result	Recommendation
Kitchen	18	Is it easy to get the most common kitchen items without climbing, bending or affecting your balance	☐Yes ☐No	Organize your kitchen so that you have easier access to the most commonly used utensils. Can be equipped with hand push wheel. Use a sturdy ladder with a broad base if you must reach high
	19	Is the light in the kitchen bright	☐Yes ☐No	The light should be bright
	20	Do you often wipe the spilled liquid off immediately	☐Yes ☐No	The spilled liquid should be wiped clean at any time
	21	Is there good ventilation to reduce the risk of blurred eyes	☐Yes ☐No	Indwelling vents, installing kitchen range hoods or exhaust fans, should be ventilated when cooking
	22	Is there a smoke alarm	☐Yes ☐No	A smoke alarm device should be installed
	23	Is there a home fire extinguisher	☐Yes ☐No	Household fire extinguishers should be provided
Living room	24	Is it easy to get up from the couch	☐Yes ☐No	Chairs that are highly suitable and have strong armrests should be used
	25	Are there any wires, furniture, and messy things in the aisle	☐Yes ☐No	Do not place telephone lines, wires, and other debris on the aisle
	26	Is the furniture placed in a suitable position so that you don't have to stretch your hands too far or bend when you open the window or take it	☐Yes ☐No	Furniture should be placed in a suitable location and the floor should be flat, non-slip and safe
	27	Are the colors of curtains and other items too close to the surrounding environment	☐Yes ☐No	Items such as curtains are as bright as possible and should be different from the surrounding environment
Bedroom	28	Are there any safety hazards in the room, such as chairs that are too high or too low, messy household items, etc.	☐Yes ☐No	Do not put anything on the floor of the bedroom. To tie the loose telephone lines and wires in the bedroom, there should be no messy items on the passage. The height of the chair should be appropriate
	29	Is there any night lighting in the room? Can you turn on the lights before getting out of bed	☐Yes ☐No	Put a light next to your bed, consider a button light or night light. It's best to keep a flashlight by your bed at night

Table B. 10 (*continued*)

Items	Number	Evaluation items	Result	Recommendation
Bedroom	30	Is there an emergency call facility in the room	☐Yes ☐No	Install an emergency pager
	31	Is it easy to get on and off	☐Yes ☐No	The height of the bed should be moderate and the hard mattress can be easily accessed. Get out of bed should be slow, sit up and stand slowly
	32	Is there a phone in the bedroom	☐Yes ☐No	In the bedroom, you should install a telephone or extension, and put it in a place where you can reach it on the bed
	33	Is the electric blanket wire secured and will not trip you? Is the button available on the bed	☐Yes ☐No	The line should be fastened and the button should be placed on the bed to reach the position
	34	Does the bedspread have a rope loop	☐Yes ☐No	There should be no ropes on the bedspread
	35	If you use crutches or walkers, are they placed where you can easily get them before you get out of bed	☐Yes ☐No	Place the crutches or the walker in a suitable place
The stairs with the ladder	36	Can you see the edge of the stairs clearly	☐Yes ☐No	Stairs and steps need additional lighting and should be bright. Use automatic switches when possible
	37	Are the lights of stairs and steps bright	☐Yes ☐No	Keep the lights bright
	38	Are there light switches up and down the stairs	☐Yes ☐No	There should be light switches above and below stairs
	39	Does the edge of each stair have non-slip mat installed	☐Yes ☐No	There must be handrails on at least one side of all stairs, the edge of each stair should be installed non-slip mat
	40	Is the stair handrail sturdy	☐Yes ☐No	Handrails must be sturdy
	41	Are the ladder and ladder stool short and firm, with the foot of the ladder covered by non-slip rubber	☐Yes ☐No	Avoid using ladders as much as possible. If needed, have someone around when using the ladder. Ladders should be maintained in good condition, preferably with handrails

Table B. 10 （*continued*）

Items	Number	Evaluation items	Result	Recommendation
Clothes with shoes	42	Do you wear shoes with non-slip soles	☐Yes ☐No	Shoes or slippers should have non-slip soles and protruding lines
	43	Do shoes have wide heels	☐Yes ☐No	Shoes should have wide round heels
	44	Do you wear street shoes outside the house instead of slippers	☐Yes ☐No	Avoid wearing only socks，loose slippers，leather-sole or other slippery-sole shoes and high heels
	45	Do clothes fit you and have no dangling cords or ruffles	☐Yes ☐No	Don't wear clothes that are too long with the possibility of tripping over it （especially pajamas）
	46	Are you sitting while putting on clothes	☐Yes ☐No	Sit down while putting on clothes; do not stand on one
legoutdoor environment	47	Are the edges of the steps clearly marked	☐Yes ☐No	The leading edge of the steps should be painted in different colors to ensure all steps are easy to see
	48	Are there self-adhesive non-slip mat at the edges of the steps	☐Yes ☐No	The edge of the steps shall be affixed with non-slip mat
	49	Do the steps have firm handrails that are easy-to-grab	☐Yes ☐No	Steps should have firm handrails that are easy to grasp
	50	Are the paths around the house in good condition	☐Yes ☐No	Keep the paths flat. Remove moss and leaves from the path. Pay extra attention when the road is wet
	51	Are the paths and entrances brightly lit at night	☐Yes ☐No	Paths and entrances should be brightly lit at night
	52	Are there grease and gasoline on the garage floors	☐Yes ☐No	Garage floors should be free of grease and gasoline
	53	Are the public places around the house maintained in good condition	☐Yes ☐No	Public places should be maintained in good condition

Table B. 11 Fall risk assessment scale

Evaluation of project	Evaluation content	Weight	Score	Evaluation of project	Evaluation content	Weight	Score
Mobility	Abnormal gait/prosthesis	3		Mental status	Delirium	3	
	Walking with assistant equipment	3			Dementia	3	
					Excitement/behavior disorder	2	
	Walking with help	3			Trance	3	

Table B. 11 （*continued*）

Evaluation of project	Evaluation content	Weight	Score	Evaluation of project	Evaluation content	Weight	Score
Self-control	Incontinence	1		Sensooy disturbance	Visually impaired	1	
	Diabetes medication	1			Hearing-impaired	1	
	Keeping catheter	1			Sensory aphasia	1	
History of falling	A history of falling	2			Other situations	1	
	Hospitalized for falling	3		Sleep	Easily wakened	1	
Medication	New drugs	1			Insomnia	1	
	Cardiovascular medication	1			Somnambulism	1	
	Blood pressure medication	1		Age	Age 80 and above	3	
					others	1	
	Sedatives and hypnotics	1		Related disease history	Neurological disease	1	
	Withdrawal treatment	1			Osteoporosis	1	
	Diabetes medication	1			History of fracture	1	
	Antiepileptic drugs	1			Low blood pressure	1	
	Anesthetics	1			Drug/alcohol withdrawal	1	
	Others	1			Anoxia	1	
				Total evaluation score：			
Assessment criteria：low risk：1~2 points；Medium risk：3~9 points；High risk：10 or above.							

Table B. 12 Morse fall assessement scale

Number	Evaluation content	Scoring	Tips	Score
1	History of falling；immediate or within 3 months	No＝0□ Yes＝25□	Ask patients and caregivers for a history of trip and fall within the past three months. Older patients may give inaccurate results due to memory loss or concerns over self-esteem	
2	Secondary diagnosis	No＝0□ Yes＝15□	Query resident's chart	
3	Ambulatory aid	Bed rest/nurse assist＝0□ Crutches/cane/walker＝15□ Furniture＝30□	Can walk on their own，or do not need to walk at all. Ask after observation（patient and caregiver）	

Table B. 12 （*continued*）

Number	Evaluation content	Scoring	Tips	Score
4	IV/Heparin Lock	No = 0□ Yes = 20□	The patient uses anesthetics, antihista-mines, antihypertensives, sedative-hyp-notics, antiepileptic drugs, laxatives, di-uretics, hypoglycemic agents, antide-pressant anti-anxiety antipsychotics	
5	Gait/Transferring	fatigue/Bed rest/Wheelchair walking = 0□ ≥ age 65/ postural? hypotension = 10□ Impaired = 20□	Patients with a normal gait or complete bed-ridden patients with weak lower limbs do not necessarily have decreased muscle strength and function. Decreased or disability of motor function of one or both limbs due to neurological impairment or bone and joint disease	
6	Mental status	Awareness of their own abili-ty = 0□ Ignorance of limitations/ Dis-order of consciousness/rest-lessness/communication bar-rier / sleep disorder = 15□	No cognitive impairment: Compliance with medical treatment, can change bad behavior due to the mission. Cognitive impairment: overconfidence, non-compliance with medical treatment, etc.	

Assessment criteria: Low risk：<25 points；Medium risk：25～45 points；High risk：>45 points.

Table B. 13 Clinical dementia rating （CDR）

Impairment	Health CDR = 0	Questionable CDR = 0.5	Mild CDR = 1	Moderate CDR = 2	Severe CDR = 3
Memory	No memory loss or slight inconstant forget-fulness	Consistent slight forgetfulness, par-tial recollection of events, "benign" forgetful-ness	Moderate memory loss; prominent forgetting for re-cent events; mem-ory impairment in-terferes with daily life	Severe memory loss; can only re-member highly fa-miliar events; re-cent events are rapidly lost	Severe mem-ory loss; only fragments re-main
Orientation	Fully oriented	Fully oriented ex-cept for slight diffi-culty with timeline	Moderate difficulty with timelines; ori-ented for a place at the examination; may have geographic dis-orientation elsewhere	Severe difficulty with timelines; usually dis-oriented to time, of-ten to place	Oriented to pe-rson only

Table B. 13（*continued*）

Impairment	Health CDR = 0	Questionable CDR = 0.5	Mild CDR = 1	Moderate CDR = 2	Severe CDR = 3
Judgment and problem solving	Solves everydayproblems and handles business and financial affairs well；have good judgment in relation to past performance	Slight impairment in solving problems，recognizing the similarities and differences between objects	Moderate difficulty in handling problems, identifying similarities and differences between tasks，and often maintaining social judgment	Severely impaired in handling problems，similarities，and differences；social judgment usually impaired	Be unable to make judgments or solve problems
Community affairs	Work，shop，volunteer and socialize independently as usual	Slight impairment in these activities	Be unable to function independently at these activities although may still be engaged in some，appears normal to casual inspection	No desire to go outside individually Appears well enough to be taken to functions outside a family home	Appears too ill to be taken to functions outside a family home
Home and Hobbies	Life at home，hobbies，and intellectual interests well maintained	Life at home，hobbies，and intellectualinterests slightlyimpaired	Mild but definite impairment of function at home，more difficult chores abandoned，more complicated hobbies and interests abandoned	Only simple chores preserved，very restricted interests，poorly maintained	No significant function at home
Personal care	Fully capable of self-care	Require others' supervisions	Require others' assistance to put on clothes, hygiene, and other personal stuff	Require assistance in dressing, hygiene, keeping of personal effects loss of bladder control	Requires much help with personal care，frequent incontinence

Description：Scores（of 0.5、1、2 or 3）apply when damage is only caused by congnitive impairments.

Table B.14 Confusion assessment method（CAM）

Number	Evaluation of project	Evaluation content	Scoring	Score
1	Acute onset and fluctuating course	1a. Is there evidence of an acute change in the patient's mental status compared to usual?	No = 0 Yes = 1	
		1b. Did these abnormal behaviors fluctuate during the day （which means the symptoms tend to come and go or increase and decrease in severity）?	No = 0 Yes = 12	
2	Inattention	2. Did the patient have difficulty keeping their focus （for example, being easily distracted or having difficulty keeping track of what was being said）?	No = 0 Yes = 1	
3	Disorganized thinking	3. Was the patient's thinking disorganized or incoherent, such as rambling or irrelevant conversation, unclear or illogical flow of ideas, or unpredictable changes on subjects from one to another?	No = 0 Yes = 1	
4	Altered consciousness	4. Overall, how would you rate this patient's level of consciousness? Overly alerted, hypersomnia, numb or unconscious?	No = 0 Yes = 1	
Description: Delirium occurs when 1a,1b and 2 are both "yes" and either 3 or 4 are "yes".				

Table B.15 Mini nutritional assessment（MNA）

Number	Evaluation of project	Scoring	Score
1	Has food intake declined over the past 3 months due to loss of appetite, digestive problems, chewing or swallowing difficulties?	0 = severe decrease in food intake 1 = moderate decrease in food intake 2 = no decrease in food intake	
2	Weight loss during the last 3 months	0 = weight loss greater than 3 kg （6.6 lbs） 1 = does not know 2 = weight loss between 1 and 3 kg （2.2 and 6.6 lbs） 3 = no weight loss	
3	Mobility	0 = bed or chair bound 1 = able to get out of bed / chair but does not go out 2 = goes out	
4	Has suffered psychological stress or acute disease in the past 3 months?	0 = yes 2 = no	
5	Neuropsychological problems	0 = severe dementia or depression 1 = mild dementia 2 = no psychological problems	

Table B. 15 （continued）

Number	Evaluation of project	Scoring	Score
6	Body mass index（BMI）/（kg /m²）	0 = BMI less than 19 1 = 19≤BMI< 21 2 = 21≤BMI< 23 3 = BMI≥ 23	

Screening score（Total score: 14 points）:≥12 points,Normal nutritional status. There is no need to complete the assessment.

≤11 points,At risk of malnutrition,continue with the assessment to gain a Malnutrition Indicator Score

Number	Evaluation of project	Scoring	Score
7	Live independently （not in a nursing home or hospital）	0 = No 1 = Yes	
8	Take more than 3 prescription drugs per day	0 = Yes 1 = No	
9	Pressure sores or skin ulcers	0 = Yes 1 = No	
10	How many full meals does the patient eat daily?	0 = 1 meal 1 = 2 meals 2 = 3 meals	
11	Selected consumption markers for protein intake: At least one serving of dairy products(milk, yogurt) per day （yes/no） Two or more servings of legumes or eggs per week(yes/no) Meat, fish or poultry every day(yes/no)	0 = if 0 or 1 yes 0. 5 = if 2 yes 1 = if 3 yes	
12	Consume two or more servings of fruit or vegetables per day?	0 = No 1 = Yes	
13	How much fluid （water, juice, coffee, tea, milk,etc. ） is consumed per day?	0 = less than 3 cups 0. 5 = 3 to 5 cups 1 = more than 5 cups	
14	Mode of feeding	0 = unable to eat without assistance 1 = self-fed with some difficulty 2 = self-fed without any problem	
15	Self-evaluation of nutritional status	0 = views the self as being malnourished 1 = is uncertain of nutritional state 2 = views the self as having no nutritional problem	
16	What do patients think of their health compared to their peers?	0 = bad 0. 5 = unaware 1 = just as good 2 = better	

Table B. 15（continued）

Number	Evaluation of project	Scoring	Score
17	Upper-arm circumference MAC（cm）	0 = MAC＜21 0.5 = 21≤MAC＜22 1 = MAC≥22	
18	Calf girth CC（cm）	0 = CC＜31　1 = CC≥31	

Evaluation Results：
Screening Project Score：
Evaluation item score（up to 16 points）：
Total score：

Malnutrition guidance：17～23.5 points：There is a risk of malnutrition；＜17 points：The patient is malnourished.

Table B. 16　Nutritional risk screening 2002（NRS2002）

Base situation	Name		Admission number	
	Sex		Lesion	
	Age		Bed number	
	Height		Weight（kg）	
	Body mass index（BMI）		Protein（g/L）	
	Clinical diagnosis			

	Type and name of a disease	Fraction	score
Disease condition	Patients with pelvic fractures or chronic diseases have the following diseases：liver cirrhosis, chronic obstructive pulmonary disease, long-term dialysis, diabetic tumors	1	
	Major abdominal surgery, stroke, severe pneumonia, hematological tumors	2	
	Craniocerebral injury, bone marrow suppression, and patient care（APACHE＞10 points）	3	

	Nutritional status indicators（single choice）	Fraction	score
Nutriture	Normal nutritional status	0	
	Weight loss ＞ 5% in 3 months or less in the last week（compared with requirements）20%～50%	1	
	Weight loss ＞ 5 % or BMI 18.5～20.5 or 50%～75% reduction in food intake in the last week（compared with requirements）within 2 months	2	
	Weight loss ＞ 5% in 1 month（or ＞ 15% in 3 months）or BMI ＜ 18.5（or serum albumin ＜ 35g/L）or 70%～100% less intake in the last week（compared with residual requirements）	3	
Age	Age ≥ 70 years old plus 1 point	1	

The total score of nutritional risk：screening

Assessment and intervention recommendations：
The total score of ≥ 3.0, the patient has the risk of malnutrition and needs nutritional support treatment.
Total score ＜ 3.0：if the patient will undergo major surgery, the nutritional status of the patient will be reassessed weekly.

Table B.17 Geriatric depression scale-5（GDS-5）

Ask the subject about the past week：			
Number	Evaluation content	Grade	Score
1	Are you basically satisfied with your life?	yes = 0；no = 1	
2	Do you often get bored?	yes = 1；no = 0	
3	Do you often feel that no matter what you do, it is useless?	yes = 1；no = 0	
4	Do you prefer to stay at home rather than go out and do new things?	yes = 1；no = 0	
5	Do you think your life is worthless now?	yes = 1；no = 0	
Total evaluation score：			
Evaluation criteria： Less than 2 points, normal； ≥ 2 points, suspected depression			

Table B.18 Geriatric depression scale-15（GDS-15）

Ask the subject about the past week.			
Number	Evaluation content	Grade	Score
1	Are you basically satisfied with your life?	yes = 0；no = 1	
2	Do you often get bored?	yes = 1；no = 0	
3	Do you often feel that no matter what you do, it is useless?	yes = 1；no = 0	
4	Do you prefer to stay at home rather than go out and do new things?	yes = 1；no = 0	
5	Do you feel that your life is worthless now?	yes = 1；no = 0	
6	Do you reduce a lot of activities and hobbies?	yes = 1；no = 0	
7	Do you think your life is empty?	yes = 1；no = 0	
8	Are you in good spirits most of the time?	yes = 0；no = 1	
9	Are you afraid that something unfortunate will happen to you?	yes = 1；no = 0	
10	Do you feel happy most of the time?	yes = 0；no = 1	
11	Do you think you have more memory problems than most people?	yes = 1；no = 0	
12	Do you think "still alive" is a good thing?	yes = 0；no = 1	
13	Do you feel energetic?	yes = 0；no = 1	
14	Do you think your current situation is hopeless?	yes = 1；no = 0	
15	Do you think most people are happier than you?	yes = 1；no = 0	
Total evaluation score：			
Evaluation criteria： 1 ≤ 4 points, regardless of depression； 5 ≤ 9 points, possible depression； ≥ 10, depression.			

Table B.19 Assessment form of skin risk factors (Braden scale)

Number	Evaluation project	Scoring content and scoring criteria				Score
		1	2	3	4	
1	Consciousness condition	Complete coma	Coma but response to pain.	Awake, but some of the senses are damaged	Awake and normal	
2	Cleaning condition	Incontinence dampness	Incontinence, change every day≤3	Incontinence, every change	Dry, clean	
3	Mobility	Completely restricted immobility	Most of them don't move	Partial restriction	No restriction	
4	Capacity for action	Strict bed rest	Sitting posture only (wheelchair)	Get out of bed a lot	Get out of bed freely	
5	Diet condition	Jejunitas	Intake less than 1 200 calories per day	The intake can reach more than one and a half of the required amount, and tube feeding or total parenteral nutrition (TPN) can achieve most of the nutritional needs	Intake ≥ required	
6	Friction force and shear force	Something the matter	There are potential problems.	No problem		
Total evaluation score(Score range 6 ～ 23)						
Evaluation criteria: 15 points ～18 points, low risk; 13 points ～14 points, medium risk; 10 points ～12 points, high risk; ≤ 9 points, very high risk.						

Bibliography

［1］ MZ/T 001—2013 Ability assessment for the elderly

［2］ Basic Standards of Nursing Homes,National Health and Family Planning Commission of the People's Republic of China〔2011〕No. 21.

［3］ Chinese catalog of rehabilitation aids , 2014.

［4］ National standards and norms for hospital informatization construction（trial）. Planning and Information Department of National Health and Health Commission and Statistical Information Center of National Health and Health Commission, April 2018.

［5］ Song huiping, Chen zheng. Geriatric friendly hospital. Chinese journal of gerontology. 2016,8（35）:1018-1021.

［6］ Song yuetao, Chen zheng, Gao maolong , et al. Interpretation of the standards of elderly-friendly hospitals in Beijing. Chinese journal of geriatric care medicine, 2008,16（3）:11-15.

［7］ Zhou yanming , et al. Architectural details of nursing facilities . Design and interpretation of Elderly Care Facility. China Architecture and Building Press.

［8］ Song yuetao, Jin zhe, Gao maolong, et al. Basic standards and service specifications for comprehensive assessment of the elderly in medical service institutions（trial）. Chinese geriatric healthcare medicine, 2008,16(3):3-10.

［9］ Song yuetao. Comprehensive geriatric assessment（second edition）. Beijing: China union medical university press, 2019.

［10］ World Health Organization. Global Age-friendly Cities: A Guide. 2007. http://www. who. int/kobe_centre/publications/age_friendly_cities_guide/en/

［11］ World Health Organization. WHO age-friendly environments, programme. http://www. who. int/ageing/age_friendly_cities/en/index. html

［12］ World Health Organization. Age-friendly Primary Health Care Centres Toolkit. http://www. who. int/ageing/publications/Age-Friendly-PHC-Centre-toolkitDec08. pdf

［13］ World Health Organization. Active Aging: Towards Age-friendly Primary Health Care. http://www. who. int/hpr/ageing

［14］ Health Promotion Administration, Ministry of Health and Welfare: Age-friendly Hospitals and

Health Services Recognition Self-assessment. Manual http://www. hpa. gov. tw/BHPNet/Web/ HealthTopic/TopicArticle. aspx

[15]　Regional Geriatric Program of Toronto，Senior Friendly Hospitals，A Toolkit for Senior Friendly Hospitals. RGP,2011. http://senior friendly hospitals. ca.

ICS 67.040
X 80

团　体　标　准

T/CGSS 004—2019

适老营养配方食品通则

General rules for nutrition formula food for the elderly

2019-04-23 发布

2019-04-23 实施

中国老年医学学会　发　布

75

前　　言

本标准按照 GB/T 1.1—2009 给出的规则起草。

本标准由中国老年医学学会科技成果转化工作委员会、中国老年医学学会营养与食品安全分会提出。

本标准由中国老年医学学会归口。

本标准起草单位:中国老年医学学会科技成果转化工作委员会、中国老年医学学会营养与食品安全分会、中润利华(北京)营养科技有限公司、杭州纽曲星生物科技有限公司、解放军总医院国家老年疾病临床医学研究中心、四川大学华西医院、北京协和医院、广西医科大学第一附属医院、华中科技大学附属同济医院、陆军军医大学大坪医院、中国人民解放军联勤保障部队第 903 医院、南方医科大学深圳医院、江苏省人民医院、中国医科大学附属医院、贵阳医学院附属医院、河北省人民医院。

本标准主要起草人:胡雯、程志、于康、裴耀东、刘春源、张勇胜、姚颖、缪明永、许红霞、尤祥妹、郑延松、吴砚荣、朱翠凤、马向华、胡怀东、施万英、杨大刚、刘庆春、张晓伟、饶志勇、柳园、孙静、刘英华、蒋希乐、于凤梅、景小凡、李晶晶、石磊、程懿、税启航、吴琦、林根、陈水超、田文。

适老营养配方食品通则

1 范围

本标准规定了适老营养配方食品的术语和定义、适老营养配方食品分类、技术要求、安全性要求、食品添加剂和营养强化剂、标签。

本标准适用于老年人群的营养配方食品。

2 规范性引用文件

下列文件对于本文件的应用是必不可少的。凡是注日期的引用文件,仅注日期的版本适用于本文件。凡是不注日期的引用文件,其最新版本(包括所有的修改单)适用于本文件。

GB 2760 食品安全国家标准 食品添加剂使用标准

GB 2761 食品安全国家标准 食品中真菌毒素限量

GB 2762 食品安全国家标准 食品中污染物限量

GB 4789.1 食品安全国家标准 食品微生物学检验 总则

GB 4789.2 食品安全国家标准 食品微生物学检验 菌落总数测定

GB 4789.3 食品安全国家标准 食品微生物学检验 大肠菌群计数

GB 4789.4 食品安全国家标准 食品微生物学检验 沙门氏菌检验

GB 4789.10 食品安全国家标准 食品微生物学检验 金黄色葡萄球菌检验

GB 4789.34 食品安全国家标准 食品微生物学检验 双歧杆菌检验

GB 4789.35 食品安全国家标准 食品微生物学检验 乳酸菌检验

GB 5009.5 食品安全国家标准 食品中蛋白质的测定

GB 5009.11 食品国家安全标准 食品中总砷及无机砷的测定

GB 5009.12 食品安全国家标准 食品中铅的测定

GB 5009.13 食品安全国家标准 食品中铜的测定

GB 5009.14 食品安全国家标准 食品中锌的测定

GB 5009.22 食品安全国家标准 食品中黄曲霉毒素 B 族和 G 族的测定

GB 5009.24 食品安全国家标准 食品中黄曲霉毒素 M 族的测定

GB 5009.33 食品安全国家标准 食品中亚硝酸盐与硝酸盐的测定

GB 5009.82 食品安全国家标准 食品中维生素 A、D、E 的测定

GB 5009.84 食品安全国家标准 食品中维生素 B_1 的测定

GB 5009.85 食品安全国家标准 食品中维生素 B_2 的测定

GB 5009.86 食品安全国家标准 食品中抗坏血酸的测定

GB 5009.87 食品安全国家标准 食品中磷的测定

GB 5009.88 食品安全国家标准 食品中膳食纤维的测定

GB 5009.89 食品安全国家标准 食品中烟酸和烟酰胺的测定

GB 5009.90 食品安全国家标准 食品中铁的测定

GB 5009.91 食品安全国家标准 食品中钾、钠的测定

GB 5009.92 食品安全国家标准 食品中钙的测定

GB 5009.93　食品安全国家标准　食品中硒的测定

GB 5009.154　食品安全国家标准　食品中维生素 B$_6$ 的测定

GB 5009.168　食品安全国家标准　食品中脂肪酸的测定

GB 5009.210　食品安全国家标准　食品中泛酸的测定

GB 5009.211　食品安全国家标准　食品中叶酸的测定

GB 5009.241　食品安全国家标准　食品中镁的测定

GB 5009.242　食品安全国家标准　食品中锰的测定

GB 5413.14　食品安全国家标准　婴幼儿食品和乳品中维生素 B$_{12}$ 的测定

GB 7718　食品安全国家标准　预包装食品标签通则

GB 13432　食品安全国家标准　预包装特殊膳食用食品标签

GB 14880　食品安全国家标准　食品营养强化剂使用标准

GB/Z 21922　食品营养成分基本术语

GB/T 22492　大豆肽粉

GB 28050　食品安全国家标准　预包装食品营养标签通则

GB 29921　食品安全国家标准　食品中致病菌限量

GB 31645　食品安全国家标准　胶原蛋白肽

3　术语和定义

下列术语和定义适用于本文件。

3.1

营养素　nutrient

食物中具有特定生理作用,能维持机体生长、发育、活动、生殖以及正常代谢所需的物质,缺少这些物质,将导致机体发生相应的生化或生理学的不良变化。包括蛋白质、脂肪、碳水化合物、矿物质、维生素五大类。

［GB/Z 21922—2008 术语和定义 2.1.2］

3.2

适老营养配方食品　nutrition formula food for the elderly

根据老年人的生理特点和营养需求,调整某一种或多种营养素含量及比例,改善食物质地,添加(或不添加)益生菌和(或)益生元,配制加工的预包装食品。

4　适老营养配方食品分类

4.1　按调整的营养素分类:

　　a)　蛋白质类;

　　b)　脂肪类;

　　c)　碳水化合物类;

　　d)　维生素类;

　　e)　矿物质类。

4.2　按质地分类:

　　a)　流质型;

　　b)　半流质型;

　　c)　软食型;

　　d)　粉末型。

4.3 其他类别

添加益生菌、益生元类。

5 技术要求

5.1 基本要求

5.1.1 适老营养配方应以老年医学或营养学的研究结果为依据,针对老年人因各种原因营养摄入不足而引起的营养不良,进行营养素补充。

5.1.2 适老营养配方食品应以满足老年人群特定需求为首要条件。

5.2 原料要求

适老营养配方食品的原料应符合相应的国家标准和(或)相关规定,不应使用可能危害老年人群健康的物质。

5.3 感官指标要求

适老营养配方食品的外观、色泽、味道、气味、质地、口感应符合相应产品的特性,易咀嚼、易吞咽,不应有肉眼可见的外来异物。

5.4 技术特征及指标要求

5.4.1 食品类别性状特征

食品类别性状特征及检测方法见表1。

表1 食品类别性状特征及检测方法

类 型	性状特征	检测方法
流质型	含渣极少、结构均匀的液态食物,用吸管可轻松吸取	方法一:测试样品流经10 mmL注射器,10 s后注射器的残留量较少。 方法二:测试样品能够快速地从侧倾汤勺中流出
半流质型	结构均匀、顺滑,吸管难以吸食	测试样品需要轻叩汤勺才能滑落移出,可在汤勺上留下残余
软食型	结构松软、湿润,可用舌头和上颚碾碎或可轻松咀嚼的食物,可含有少量颗粒,不含硬块	测试样品可用手指轻松压扁,在餐盘上可成团状或缓慢塌陷
粉末型[a]	小于1 mm的分散性可溶食品小颗粒或速溶颗粒	100%通过15 μm筛网

[a] 参考《材料科学技术名词》第一版,2011。

5.4.2 营养指标

5.4.2.1 根据老年人的生理特点和营养需求,不同的营养配方应添加必要的营养素。应添加必要的营养素种类及指标见表2。

表 2　必要的营养素种类及指标

营养素分类	营养素名称	指标(100 g 固态物,液态物以所含 100 g 固态物计算)	检验方法
蛋白质类	蛋白质水解物	≥30%[a]	GB 5009.5[a] GB/T 22492 GB 31645
	优质蛋白质	≥50%[b]	—
	谷氨酰胺	10%～20%[b]	—
脂肪类	n-3 脂肪酸[c]	供能比 0.5%～2%	GB 5009.168
	n-6 脂肪酸[d]	供能比 2.5%～9%	GB 5009.168
	反式脂肪酸	0	GB 5009.168
碳水化合物类	碳水化合物	供能比≥50%	GB/Z 21922
	膳食纤维(g)	5～10.8	GB 5009.88
维生素类		见表 4	
矿物质类		见表 4	

注:上述营养素可根据需要添加一种或多种。

[a] 食品中总蛋白质含量测定标准。

[b] 占总蛋白质的含量比例。

[c] 其中 α-亚麻酸供能比≥0.5%。

[d] 其中亚油酸供能比≥2%。

5.4.2.2　根据老年人的生理特点和营养需求,宜添加一种或多种益生菌和益生元,益生菌、益生元的种类及指标见表 3。

表 3　益生菌、益生元种类及指标

类　别	名　称	指　标	检验方法
益生菌类	青春双歧杆菌、动物双歧杆菌(乳双歧杆菌)、两歧双歧杆菌、短双歧杆菌、婴儿双歧杆菌、长双歧杆菌、嗜酸乳杆菌、干酪乳杆菌、卷曲乳杆菌、发酵乳杆菌、格氏乳杆菌、瑞士乳杆菌、约氏乳杆菌、副干酪乳杆菌、植物乳杆菌、罗伊氏乳杆菌、鼠李糖乳杆菌、唾液乳杆菌	≥10^7 CFU/g(mL)	GB 4789.34 GB 4789.35
益生元类	低聚果糖、低聚异麦芽糖、菊粉、水苏糖等	5～15 g/100 g 固态物	GB 5009.88

5.4.2.3　适老营养配方食品宜添加营养素的种类和添加量见表 4。

表 4　营养素的种类和添加量

营养素名称(单位)	指标(100 g固态物,液态物以所含100 g固态物计算)		检验方法
	最小值	最大值	
维生素 A(μg RE)	300	900	GB 5009.82
维生素 D(μg)	6.3	12.5	GB 5009.82
维生素 E(mgα-TE)	10	31	GB 5009.82
维生素 B_1(mg)	0.9	2.2	GB 5009.84
维生素 B_2(mg)	0.9	2.2	GB 5009.85
维生素 B_6(mg)	0.7	2.2	GB 5009.154
维生素 B_{12}(μg)	1	6.6	GB 5413.14
烟酸(烟酰胺)(mg)	11	33	GB 5009.89
叶酸(μg)	60	600	GB 5009.211
泛酸(mg)	2.2	8	GB 5009.210
维生素 C(mg)	100	225	GB 5009.86
钠(mg)	330	N.S.	GB 5009.91
钾(mg)	450	N.S.	GB 5009.91
铜(μg)	300	750	GB 5009.13
镁(mg)	130	210	GB 5009.241
铁(mg)	6	20	GB 5009.90
锌(mg)	6	18	GB 5009.14
锰(μg)	30	430	GB 5009.242
钙(mg)	250	1 000	GB 5009.92
磷(mg)	196	700	GB 5009.87
硒(μg)	14	28	GB 5009.93

6　安全性要求

6.1　污染物限量

食品中污染物限量应符合 GB 2762 中相同或相近产品类别的要求,无相应类属食品的应符合表5的要求。

表5 污染物限量

污染物名称	限量（mg/kg）	检验方法
铅	0.5	GB 5009.12
总砷（As）[a]	1.0	GB 5009.11
硝酸盐(以 NaNO$_3$ 计)[b]	100	GB 5009.33
亚硝酸盐(以 NaNO$_2$ 计)[c]	2.0	

[a] 液态产品的总砷≤0.2 mg/kg。

[b] 不适用于添加蔬菜和水果的产品。

[c] 仅适用于乳基产品(不含豆类成分)。

6.2 真菌毒素限量

真菌毒素限量应符合表6的要求。

表6 真菌毒素限量

真菌毒素名称	限量(μg/kg)	检验方法
黄曲霉毒素 B$_1$[a]	0.5	GB 5009.22
黄曲霉毒素 M$_1$[b]	0.5	GB 5009.24

[a] 仅适用于以豆类及大豆蛋白制品为主要原料的产品。

[b] 仅适用于以乳类及乳蛋白制品为主要原料的产品。

6.3 微生物限量

微生物限量应符合 GB 29921 中相应类属食品的要求。无相应类属食品规定的应符合表7的要求。

表7 微生物限量

项 目	采样方案[a] 及限量(若非指定,均以 CFU/g 表示)				检验方法
	n	c	m	M	
菌落总数[b]	5	2	1 000	10 000	GB 4789.2
大肠菌群	5	2	10	100	GB 4789.3 平板计数法
沙门氏菌	5	0	0/25 g	—	GB 4789.4
金黄色葡萄球菌	5	2	10	100	GB 4789.10 平板计数法

[a] 样品的分析及处理按 GB 4789.1 执行。

[b] 不适用于添加活性益生菌的活菌数≥10^7 CFU/g 的产品。

7 食品添加剂和营养强化剂

7.1 食品添加剂的使用应符合 GB 2760 的要求。

7.2 营养强化剂的使用应符合 GB 14880 的规定。

7.3 食品添加剂和营养强化剂的质量规格应符合相应的国家及行业标准和有关规定。

8 标签

8.1 适老营养配方食品标签应符合 GB 7718、GB 13432、GB 28050 的规定。

8.2 标签应标注为"适老营养配方食品",并根据营养素和(或)食品质地的具体类别标明,如"适老营养配方食品(蛋白质类)""适老营养配方食品(复配型)""适老营养配方食品(流质型)"。

8.3 有关适老营养配方食品食用、配制指导说明及图解、贮存条件应在标签上明确说明。

8.4 标签应提示"对配料表中成分有过敏的人谨慎使用"或类似用语。

8.5 标签应对配制不当和使用不当可能引起的健康危害给予警示说明。

———————

ICS 67.040

X 80

Social Organization Standard

T/CGSS 004—2019

General rules for nutritional formula food for the elderly

适老营养配方食品通则

（*English Translation*）

Issue date：2019-04-23

Implementation date：2019-04-23

Issued by Chinese Geriatrics Society

Foreword

This standard was drafted in accordance with the rules given in GB/T 1. 1—2009.

This standard was proposed by Transformation of Scientific and Technological Achievements Committee of Chinese Geriatrics Society and Nutrition and Food Safety Branch of Chinese Geriatrics Society.

This standard was prepared by Chinese Geriatrics Society.

This standard was drafted by Transformation of Scientific and Technological Achievements Committee of Chinese Geriatrics Society, Nutrition and Food Safety Branch of Chinese Geriatrics Society, Zhongrunlihua (Beijing) Nutrition Technology Co. , Ltd, Hangzhou Nutrition Biotechnology Co. , Ltd, National Clinical Research Center of Geriatrics Disease (Chinese PLA General Hospital), West China Hospital of Sichuan University, Peking Union Medical College Hospital, the First Affiliated Hospital of Guangxi Medical University, Tongji Medical College of Huazhong University of Science and Technology, Daping Hospital of Army Medical University, 903rd Hospital of PLA Joint Logistics Support Force, Shenzhen Hospital of Southern Medical University, Jiangsu Province Hospital, the First Affiliated Hospital of China Medical University, the Affiliated Hospital of Guizhou Medical University and Hebei General Hospital.

The main drafters of this standard were Wen Hu, Zhi Cheng, Kang Yu, Yaodong Qiu, Chunyuan Liu, Yongsheng Zhang, Ying Yao, Mingyong Miao, Hongxia Xu, Xiangmei You, Yansong Zheng, Yanrong Wu, Cuifeng Zhu, Xianghua Ma, Huaidong Hu, Wanying Shi, Dagang Yang, QingchunLiu, Xiaowei Zhang, Zhiyong Rao, Yuan Liu, Jing Sun, Yinghua Liu, Xile Jiang, Fengmei Yu, Xiaofan Jing, Jingjing Li, Lei Shi, Yi Cheng, Qihang Shui, Qi Wu, Gen Lin, Shuichao Chen and Wen Tian.

General rules for nutritional formula food for the elderly

1 Scope

This standard specifies classification, technical requirements, safety requirements, food additives and nutritional fortification substances and labeling of nutritional formula food for theelderly.

This standard is applicable to nutritional formula food for the elderly.

2 Normative references

The following referenced documents are indispensable for the application of this document. For dated references, only the edition cited applies. For undated references, the latest edition of the referenced document (including any amendments) applies.

GB 2760   National food safety standard—Uses of food additives

GB 2761   National food safety standard—Maximum levels of mycotoxins

GB 2762   National food safety standard—Limits of contaminants in foods

GB 4789.1   National food safety standard—Food microbiological examination—General rules

GB 4789.2   National food safety standard—Food microbiological examination—Aerobic plate count

GB 4789.3   National food safety standard—Food microbiological examination—Enumeration of coliforms

GB 4789.4   National food safety standard—Food microbiological examination—Salmonella

GB 4789.10   National food safety standard—Food microbiological examination—Staphylococcus Aureus

GB 4789.34   National food safety standard—Food microbiological examination—Bifidobacterial

GB 4789.35   National food safety standard—Food microbiological examination—Lactobacillus

GB 5009. 5   National food safety standard—Determination of protein in foods

GB 5009. 11   National food safety standard—Determination of total Arsenic in foods

GB 5009. 12   National food safety standard—Determination of lead in foods

GB 5009. 13   National food safety standard—Determination of copper in foods

GB 5009. 14   National food safety standard—Determination of zinc in foods

GB 5009. 22   National food safety standard—Determination of B-group and G-groupaflatoxin in foods

GB 5009. 24   National food safety standard—Determination of M-group aflatoxin in foods

GB 5009. 33   National food safety standard—Determination of nitrite and nitrates in foods

GB 5009. 82   National food safety standard—Determination of vitamins A,D and E in foods

GB 5009. 84   National food safety standard—Determination of vitamin B_1 in foods

GB 5009. 85   National food safety standard—Determination of vitamin B_2 in foods

GB 5009. 86   National Food safety standard—Determination of ascorbic acid in foods

GB 5009. 87   National food safety standard—Determination ofphosphorus in foods

GB 5009. 88   National food safety standard—Determination of dietary fiber in foods

GB 5009. 89   National food safety standard—Determination of niacin and niacinamide in foods

GB 5009. 90   National food safety standard—Determination of iron in foods

GB 5009. 91   National food safety standard—Determination of potassium and sodium in foods

GB 5009. 92   National food safety standard—Determination of calcium in foods

GB 5009. 93   National food safety standard—Determination of selenium in foods

GB 5009. 154   National food safety standard—Determination of vitamin B_6 in foods

GB 5009. 168   National food safety standard—Determination of fatty acids in foods

GB 5009. 210   National food safety standard—Determination of pantothenic acid in foods

GB 5009. 211   National food safety standard—Determination of folic acid in foods

GB 5009. 241   National food safety standard—Determination of magnesium in foods

GB 5009. 242   National food safety standard—Determination of manganese in foods

GB 5413. 14   National food safety standard—Determination of vitamin B_{12} in baby foods and dairy products

GB 7718   National food safety standard—General rules of the labeling of prepackaged foods

GB 13432   National food safety standard—Labeling of prepackaged foods forspecial dietary uses

GB 14880   National food safety standard—Usage of nutrition enrichment

GB/Z 21922   Fundamental terminology and definitions of nutritional components in foods

GB/T 22492   Soy peptides powder

GB 28050   National food safety standard—Nutritional labeling for prepackaged food

GB 29921   National food safety standard—Maximum levels of pathogens in foods

GB 31645   National food safety standard—Collagen peptides

3   Terms and definitions

For the purposes of this document, the following terms and definitions apply.

3. 1
nutrient

substances in foods whichhave specific physiological effects in providing nourishment essentials for growth and maintenance of life, including development, activity, reproduction and metabolism; the lack of these substances will lead to corresponding physiological and biochemical adverse changes in human body; include protein, fat, carbohydrates, minerals and vitamins

[GB/Z 21922—2008, definition 2. 1. 2]

3.2
nutritional formula food for the elderly

a manufactured food formulated and produced designed to meet the nutritional needs of the elderly based on the physiological characteristics of this population by adjusting the proportion of onenutrient or more nutrients, with improved food texture, with or without additional probiotics and/or prebiotics

4 Classification of nutritional formula food for elderly

4.1 Classified by nutrient adjustment:

a) Proteins.

b) Fats.

c) Carbohydrates.

d) Vitamins.

e) Minerals.

4.2 Classified by texture:

a) Fluid type.

b) Semi-fluid type.

c) Soft food type.

d) Powder type.

4.3 other categories

additive probiotics and prebiotics.

5 Technical requirements

5.1 Basic requirements

5.1.1 The formula shall be created based on the research results of geriatrics or nutritional studies. It is designed for the elderly suffering from malnutrition due to insufficient intake for various reasons.

5.1.2   The first condition of nutritional formula food for the elderly shall be designed to meet the special nutritional needs of the elderly.

5.2   Raw material requirements

The raw materials of nutritional formula food for the elderly shall meet national standards and/or relevant regulations. Any substances that may harm human health shall not be permitted.

5.3   Sensory index

The appearance,color,taste,smell,and texture shall meet the general standards of similar food products that are easy to chew and swallow and without any visible foreign contamination.

5.4   Technical features and indicators

5.4.1   Characteristics of different food types

See Table 1 for characteristics of different food types.

Table 1   Characteristics of different food types and test methods

Type	Characteristics	Test method
Fluid type	Little pulp, consistent texture and can be consumed easily by using straws	Method 1: Let the test sample flow out of a 10 mL syringe, it is classified as liquid if there are little residues left in the syringe after 10 s. Method 2: It is qualified as liquid if the test sample flows out of the inclined spoon quickly
Semi-fluid type	Consistent texture, smooth, difficult to be consumed by using straws	It is qualified as semi-fluid if a spoonful of test sample can slide by tapping the spoon and leave some residues on the spoon
Soft food type	Soft, moist, ground easily or smashed by gum and tongue with no or very little chewing. It may contain small particles	It is classified as soft food if the test sample can be smashed easily with fingers, may form into a ball shape or slowly collapse on a dinner plate
Powder type[a]	Small, dispersible, and soluble food particles or instant soluble particles with diameters less than 1 mm	It is classified as powder if the test sample can completely pass through a 15-mesh screen
[a] Refer to the terms defined in first edition of *Materials Science and Technology*,2011.		

5.4.2   Nutritional indicators

5.4.2.1   According to the physiological characteristics and nutritional needs of the elderly, essential nutrients shall be added to nutritional formulas. The types and nutrition indicators of essential nutrients are shown in Table 2.

Table 2 Categories and indicators of essential nutrients

Category	Sub-category	Standards (Serving size :100 g solid food, or 100 g solid content of liquid food)	Test method
Proteins	protein hydrolysate	≥30%[a]	GB 5009. 5[a] GB/T 22492 GB 31645
	high-quality proteins	≥50%[b]	—
	glutamine	10%～20%[b]	—
Fats	n-3 fatty acid[c]	Fat-to-energy ratio 0. 5%～2%	GB 5009. 168
	n-6 fatty acid[d]	Fat-to-energy ratio 2. 5%～9%	GB 5009. 168
	trans-fatty acids	0	GB 5009. 168
Carbohydrates	carbohydrates	Carbohydrates-to-energy ratio ≥50%	GB/Z 21922
	dietary fiber /g	5～10. 8	GB 5009. 88
Vitamins		see Table 4	
Minerals		see Table 4	

Note:One or more of these nutrients may be added as needed.

[a] Standard for determination of total protein content in foods.

[b] Percentage of total protein content.

[c] To-energy ratio of alpha-linolenic acid is required ≥0. 5%.

[d] To-energy ratio of linoleic acid is required ≥2%.

5. 4. 2. 2 According to the physiological characteristics and nutritional needs of the elderly, it is recommended to add one or more probiotics and prebiotics. The types and nutrition indicators of probiotics and prebiotics are shown in Table 3.

Table 3 Categories and indicators of probiotics and prebiotics

Category	Sub-category	Standards	Test method
Probiotics	Bifidobacterium adolescentis, Bifidobacterium animalis(Bifidobacterium lactis), Bifidobacterium bifidum, Bifidobacterium breve, Bifidobacterium infantis, Long bifidobacterium, Lactobacillus acidophilus, Lactobacillus casei, Lactobacillus crispatus, Lactobacilus fermentum, Lactobacillus gasseri, Lactobacillus helveticus, Lactobacillus johnsonii, Lactobacillus paracasei, Lactobacillus plantarum, Lactobacillus reuteri, Lactobacillus rhamnosus, Lactobacillus salivarius	$\geqslant 10^7$ CFU/g(mL)	GB 4789.34 GB 4789.35
Prebiotics	Oligosaccharide, isomaltose, inulin, stachyose, etc.	5 g/100 g~15 g/100 g in solid food	GB 5009.88

5.4.2.3 The types of nutrients in nutritional formula food for the elderly are shown in Table 4. The amount limits of nutrient additions are advised in Table 4.

Table 4 Types and amount limits of nutrients

Nutrients/unit	Limits (Serving size :100 g solid food, or 100 g solid content of liquid food)		Test method
	minimum value	maximum value	
Vitamin A/μg RE	300	900	GB 5009.82
Vitamin D/μg	6.3	12.5	GB 5009.82
Vitamin E/mg α-TE	10	31	GB 5009.82
Vitamin B_1/mg	0.9	2.2	GB 5009.84
Vitamin B_2/mg	0.9	2.2	GB 5009.85
Vitamin B_6/mg	0.7	2.2	GB 5009.154
Vitamin B_{12}/mg	1	6.6	GB 5413.14
Niacin (niacinamide) /mg	11	33	GB 5009.89
Folic acid/μg	60	600	GB 5009.211

Table 4 (*continued*)

Nutrients/unit	Limits (Serving size :100 g solid food·or 100 g solid content of liquid food)		Test method
	minimum value	maximum value	
Pantothenic acid/mg	2. 2	8	GB 5009. 210
Vitamin C/mg	100	225	GB 5009. 86
Sodium/mg	330	N. S.	GB 5009. 91
Potassium/mg	450	N. S.	GB 5009. 91
Copper/μg	300	750	GB 5009. 13
Magnesium/mg	130	210	GB 5009. 241
Iron/mg	6	20	GB 5009. 90
Zinc/mg	6	18	GB 5009. 14
Manganese/mg	30	430	GB 5009. 242
Calcium/mg	250	1 000	GB 5009. 92
Phosphorus/mg	196	700	GB 5009. 87
Selenium/μg	14	28	GB 5009. 93

6 Safety requirements

6. 1 Limits of contamination

The limits of contaminants in foods shall meet the requirements of the same or similar product category in GB 2762·and contaminants of other categories shall meet the limit requirements of Table 5.

Table 5 Limits of contaminants

Contaminant	Standards	Test method
Lead/(mg/kg)	0. 5	GB 5009. 12
Total arsenic(As)/(mg/kg)[a]	1. 0	GB 5009. 11
Nitrate(NaNO$_3$) /(mg/kg)[b]	100	GB 5009. 33
Nitrite(NaNO$_2$)/(mg/kg)[c]	2. 0	

[a] Total arsenic in liquid products should be ≤0. 2 mg/kg.

[b] Not applicable for food with vegetables and fruits.

[c] Only applicable to whey products (without soy).

6. 2 Limits of mycotoxin

The limits of mycotoxin shall meet the requirements of Table 6.

Table 6 Limits of mycotoxin

Mycotoxins	Standards	Test method
Aspertoxin B$_1$/(μg/kg)[a]	0.5	GB 5009.22
Aspertoxin M$_1$/(μg/kg)[b]	0.5	GB 5009.24
[a] Applicable for products with beans and soybean protein as main raw materials.		
[b] Applicable for products with milk and milk protein as main raw materials.		

6.3 Limits of microbes

The limits of microbes shall meet the requirements of the corresponding food categories in GB 29921, and microbe contamination of other categories shall meet the requirements in Table 7.

Table 7 Limits of microbes

Category	Sampling method[a] and limit (CFU/g if not specified)				Test method
	n	c	m	M	
Total plate count[b]	5	2	1 000	10 000	GB 4789.2
Coliform	5	2	10	100	GB 4789.3 plate count method
Salmonella	5	0	0/25 g	—	GB 4789.4
Staphylococcus aureus	5	2	10	100	GB 4789.10 plate count method
[a] Sampling and analysis method shall be in accordance with GB 4789.1.					
[b] Not applicable for products with additive viable count of live probiotics $\geqslant 10^7$ CFU/g.					

7 Food additives and nutritional fortification substances

7.1 The uses of food additives shall meet the requirements of GB 2760.

7.2 The uses of nutritional fortification substances shall meet the provisions of GB 14880.

7.3 The quality standards of food additives and nutritional fortificationsubstances shall comply with the corresponding national and industrial standards and relevant provisions.

8 Labeling

8.1 The labeling of formula food for the elderly shall comply with the provisions in GB 7718, GB 13432 and GB 28050.

8.2　The food label shall be labeled as "nutritional formula food for the elderly" and shall provide the specific category of nutrients and/or food texture, such as "nutritional formulafood for theelderly（protein formula）""nutritional formula food for theelderly（compound formula）" and "nutritional formulafood for the elderly（fluid formula）".

8.3　Instructions and diagrams for the consumption, preparation and storage conditions of nutritional formula food for the elderly shall be shown clearly on the food label.

8.4　The food label shall indicate "use with caution if you are allergic to any ingredients in the ingredients list" or include similar terms.

8.5　The food label shall have warnings of health hazards caused by improper preparation and uses.

ICS 03.080
A 20

团　体　标　准

T/CGSS 005—2019

医养结合服务机构设施设置基本要求

Basic requirements for infrastructure for service institutions of
combination of medical and senior hearlth care

2019-04-28 发布

2019-04-28 实施

中国老年医学学会　发　布

前　言

本标准按照 GB/T 1.1—2009 给出的规则起草。

本标准由中国老年医学学会医养结合管理部和标准化管理部提出。

本标准由中国老年医学学会归口。

本标准起草单位：中国老年医学学会医养结合促进委员会、解放军总医院、国家老年疾病临床研究中心（解放军总医院）、中国中元国际工程有限公司建筑环境艺术设计研究院、辽宁省沈阳中置盛京老年医院、四川省成都青城国际颐养中心、广西壮族自治区桂林信和信健康养老产业投资有限公司、山东省临沂市凯旋老年医院、沈阳市卫生健康委员会、郑州大学第五附属医院、四川省成都市第八人民医院、甘肃省第三人民医院、山西省长治市第二人民医院、山东省滨州医学院、广州市老人院。

本标准主要起草人：杨庭树、龙宗耀、焦胜强、王群、林峰、孙志军、武强、程丽红、杨长春、侯惠如、李瑶盖、徐卫华、章亚非、姜开田、郑鹏远、黄海浪、鲁丽萍、王补青、郝玉玲、刘联琦、肖联农、陈芍、李东科。

引　言

　　目前我国60岁以上人口约达2.5亿,社会老龄化、"空巢化"程度不断加深,失能、半失能老年人不断增多,养老服务供需矛盾突出。

　　党的十九大指出,人民健康是民族昌盛和国家富强的重要标志。要积极应对人口老龄化,构建养老、孝老、敬老政策体系和社会环境,推动医养结合,加快老龄事业和产业发展。十三届人大二次会议政府工作报告指出,要大力发展养老特别是社区养老服务业,改革完善医养结合政策,使老年人拥有幸福的晚年。

　　目前,我国多种多样的养老服务机构发展迅速,以医疗资源和养老资源有机协同为一体的新型医疗护理、养老照护、康复养生型的养老服务也在全国各地广泛开展。为引领、促进和规范医养结合服务机构的发展,特制定医养结合服务机构服务设施设置基本要求。

医养结合服务机构设施设置基本要求

1 范围

本标准规定了医养结合服务机构设施设备设置的基本要求。

本标准适用于医养结合服务机构。

2 规范性引用文件

下列文件对于本文件的应用是必不可少的。凡是注日期的引用文件,仅注日期的版本适用于本文件。凡是不注日期的引用文件,其最新版本(包括所有的修改单)适用于本文件。

GB 2894 安全标志及其使用导则

GB/T 10001.1 公共信息图形符号 第1部分:通用符号

GB 18466 医疗机构污水排放标准

GB/T 18883 室内空气质量标准

GB 24436 康复训练器械 安全通用要求

GB 50011 建筑抗震设计规范

GB 50016 建筑设计防火规范

GB 50019 工业建筑供暖通风与空气调节设计规范

GB 50034 建筑照明设计标准

GB 50763 无障碍设计规范

GB 51039 综合医院建筑设计规范

JGJ 450 老年人照料设施建筑设计标准

3 术语和定义

JGJ 450 界定的以及下列术语和定义适应于本文件。

3.1

医养结合服务机构 service institutions of combination of medical and senior health care

应具备医疗、养老两方面的资质,能提供医疗、养老服务和健康管理相结合的机构。

3.2

老年养护院(老年护理院) senior nursing home(geriatric nursing home)

为老年人提供日常生活照料、医疗护理、保健康复和文化娱乐等综合性服务的养老机构。

3.3

社区日间照护中心 day care center for the aged

为生活不能完全自理的老年人提供日间日常生活照料、膳食供应、基础护理、保健康复、文化娱乐和出行协助等综合性服务的机构。

3.4

养护单元 nursing unit

为实现养护职能、保证养护质量而划分的相对独立的服务分区。

3.5

护理型床位　nursing bed

在养老机构内部面向失能、失智老年人照护服务需求而设置的床位设施。

4　总则

4.1　医养结合服务机构服务应坚持以人为本,科学、合理、适用相结合的原则,设施设置应满足老人生活照料、护理康复、保健养生、精神慰藉和安宁疗护的基本需求。

4.2　医养结合服务机构养老设施要符合老年人的生理特点,适应老年人对环境的需求,做到适老、舒适和安全可靠。

4.3　医养结合服务机构医疗设置要突出养老与医疗适度结合的特点,应符合老年人常见病、慢性病的需求,设置要有利于老年人疾病治疗与慢性病康复,有利于老年人的身心健康。

5　基本要求

5.1　养老服务设施设置要求

5.1.1　建筑选址与布局

5.1.1.1　养老服务机构的选址与布局应科学合理,符合 JGJ 450 要求。

5.1.1.2　应避免处于风口、河道、松软山体等潜在地质性安全隐患旁。

5.1.1.3　宜靠近城市公共风景休闲场所,如公园、文化中心、体育健身场地,便于利用周边社会公共服务设施。

5.1.1.4　总平面内应设置供老年人休闲、健身、娱乐等活动的室内和室外活动场所,人均面积不小于 1.20 m²。

5.1.1.5　总平面内应有景观环境和园林绿化设计,绿化种植以乔灌木、花木为主,并与草地相结合。

5.1.1.6　总平面内可设置观赏水景池,但水深不宜超过 0.6 m,并应有安全提示与安全防护措施。

5.1.1.7　公共区域和活动场所应设置公共厕所、座椅、照明、遮阳和避雨设施。

5.1.1.8　公共区域和活动场所应符合 GB 50763 要求。

5.1.1.9　大型养老设施建筑内应设置理发室、商店及银行、邮局和保险代理等生活服务用房。

5.1.1.10　新建大型养老设施建筑内应设置公共停车场所,车位数按 0.1 个车位/1 个养老床位配比。

5.1.1.11　公共区域应设明显标识,图形符号与标识的使用和设置应符合 GB/T 10001.1 和 GB 2894 的要求。

5.1.2　设施建筑要求

5.1.2.1　医养结合服务机构建筑设计应符合 JGJ 450 要求。

5.1.2.2　居住房屋建筑抗震强度应符合 GB 50011 要求。

5.1.2.3　居住用房建筑防火应符合 GB 50016 要求。

5.1.2.4　老年人居住用房的净高不宜低于 2.60 m,窗户设置应日照充足,冬日满窗日照不宜小于 2 h 且通风良好。

5.1.2.5　老年人居室门净宽不应小于 1.10 m,卫生洗浴用房门净宽不应小于 0.90 m;老年人居住区走廊净宽不应小于 2.10 m;生活区走道净宽宜为 2.40 m,至少不应小于 2.10 m。

5.1.2.6　养老用房宜以低层和多层为主,二层或以上高层建筑应设置多部垂直电梯,且应为无障碍电梯,电梯应可容纳医用床、平车和担架。二层及以上高层建筑应按每 100～120 张床位设置 1 台电梯。

5.1.2.7 宜设置急救车、老人接送车及物品采购车停车场所;应设置平车、担架车及轮椅等老人运送工具用房。

5.1.2.8 车库出口宜与外界交通便捷,救护车等老人运载工具能直达老人居住区域门口。

5.1.3 室内建筑设施设置要求

5.1.3.1 给排水系统

5.1.3.1.1 养老设施热水供应应符合 GB 50019 要求,全天 24 h 供应热水,配水点出水温度宜为 40 ℃～50 ℃,应配有控温、稳压装置。

5.1.3.1.2 排水系统通畅,医疗单位排水应符合 GB 18466 要求,独立设置管道系统并集中到统一处理池进行消毒处理。

5.1.3.2 供暖与通风空调

5.1.3.2.1 严寒和寒冷地区的养老设施建筑应设集中供暖系统,供暖方式宜选用低温热水地板辐射供暖。夏热冬冷地区也应配设供暖设施。

5.1.3.2.2 养老设施室内温度应符合 GB 50019 要求,冬季供暖温度不低于 22 ℃,夏季温度不高于 28 ℃。

5.1.3.2.3 养老设施内空气质量标准应符合 GB/T 18883 要求,公用厨房、自用与公用卫生间应设置排气通风道,并安装机械排风装置,机械排风系统应具备防回流功能。

5.1.3.2.4 养老设施内的空调系统应设置分室温度控制措施。

5.1.3.2.5 养老设施建筑内的水泵和风机等产生噪声的设备,应采取减振降噪措施。

5.1.3.3 电气与照明

5.1.3.3.1 养老设施居住、活动及辅助空间照明应符合 GB 50034 要求,选用暖色节能光源,显色指数宜大于 80,眩光指数宜小于 19。

5.1.3.3.2 养老设施居住用房及公共活动用房宜设置备用照明,并宜采用自动控制方式。

5.1.3.3.3 养老设施居住用房、卫生间、走道墙面照明应符合 JGJ 450 要求,设嵌装脚灯,住房及长走廊的顶灯宜采用两地双控开关。

5.1.3.3.4 养老设施内照明控制开关应符合 JGJ 450 要求,选用宽板翘板开关。

5.1.3.3.5 养老设施内走道、楼梯间、阳台及电梯厅等应设照明灯具,走廊、楼梯应安装应急灯,均宜采用声光控开关控制。

5.1.3.3.6 养老设施内电源插座应符合 JGJ 450 要求,距地高度低于 1.8 m 时,应采用安全型电源插座。

5.1.3.3.7 养老设施居住用房、公共活动用房和公共餐厅等应设置有线电视、电话及信息网络插座。

5.1.3.3.8 养老设施供电电源应安全可靠,宜采用专线配电,供配电系统应简明清晰,供配电支线应采用暗铺设方式。

5.1.4 室内居住设施设置要求

5.1.4.1 养老机构应根据规模大小划分为一个或多个养护单元,高层建筑宜一层为一养护单元,养老院每养护单元床位数以 50～100 张为宜,老年养护院每个养护单元床位数不应大于 50 张。

5.1.4.2 养老居住用房设置应符合 JGJ 450 要求,根据床单位数量分为单人间、双人间及多人间。单间面积不小于 10 m²,双人间面积不小于 16 m²,多人间按床单位计算,每床单位平均使用面积不小于 6 m²。

5.1.4.3 养老院每间居住卧室非护理型床位数应不大于4张,护理型床位数应不大于6张,且床与床的长边间距不应小于0.80 m;床位床边距采光外墙墙面间距不应小于0.60 m;靠通道床位端部与墙面间距不小于1.05 m。

5.1.4.4 老年养护院每间居室床位数以2～4张床为宜,应不大于4张床。

5.1.4.5 社区老年日间照料中心设置应符合国家民政部《社区老年人日间照料中心建设标准》(2010)要求,老人休息室宜为每间4～8人。

5.1.4.6 应按床位数配置相同数量的床头柜和储藏柜,储藏柜位置应方便老人取放物品,供轮椅使用者使用的储藏柜高度不应大于1.60 m。

5.1.4.7 养护院老年人居住用房内除安置床单位外宜留有轮椅、平车和诊疗床回转空间,床边应留有护理、急救操作空间。

5.1.4.8 养老院老人居住用房内应设置独立卫生间,包括厕所、盥洗室和浴室。厕所应设置坐便器,浴室应为淋浴式。坐便器、盥洗台和浴室应辅设扶手装置。

5.1.4.9 介助老人居住用房内厕所、浴室平面布置应留有助厕、助浴等操作空间。

5.1.5 餐厅设施设置要求

5.1.5.1 公共餐厅的使用面积应符合JGJ 450要求。

5.1.5.2 公共餐厅宜结合养护区域分散设置,宜每一养护单元设置一个公共餐厅,应不大于50个座位,餐厅床均使用面积应不小于0.93 m²。

5.1.5.3 高层养老建筑应每层设置小型公共餐厅及配餐间。

5.1.5.4 公共餐厅应使用可移动的、牢固稳定的单人座椅。

5.1.5.5 公共餐厅布置应能满足供餐车进出、送餐到位的服务,并应为护理员留有分餐、助餐空间。当采用柜台式售饭方式时,应设有无障碍服务柜台。

5.1.5.6 配餐间可设置在公共餐厅附近,面积不小于10 m²,供照护员为入住失能老年人分配、加热、切分食物等。

5.1.5.7 厨房设置不应靠近老人居住用房,油烟排放系统应朝向空旷区域,应避免风向朝向老人居住区域。

5.1.6 文化娱乐用房设置要求

5.1.6.1 大型高层养老建筑内应在每一层设置开敞式娱乐场所,人均面积不应低于1.20 m²,应明亮、通风,适合于进行娱乐活动。

5.1.6.2 每一养护单元应设置文化活动间,用于读书读报、下棋玩牌,房间面积应不小于20 m²,房间应有良好日照和通风。

5.1.6.3 每一养护单元应设置亲情间(可作为心理咨询室),面积应不小于12 m²,设置沙发、茶几,用于老人家属探望交流。房间应有良好日照和通风。

5.1.6.4 宜设置体育健身场所,配备适宜的运动器材。

5.1.7 信息化设置要求

5.1.7.1 医养结合服务机构应按信息化管理、网络服务以及视频传输的需要,铺设线路,预留接口。

5.1.7.2 医院信息化建设应参照国家卫生健康委员会《全国医院信息化建设标准与规范(试行)》(2018)要求。

5.1.7.3 医养结合服务机构应具备远程网络会诊平台条件。

5.1.7.4 老人居住用房内应设有线电视、电话及室内移动通信功能。

5.1.8 特殊安全设施设置要求

5.1.8.1 建筑平面内出入口、通道、走廊和房间门口无障碍通道设计应符合 GB 50763 规定。

5.1.8.2 低层养老建筑楼梯踏步前缘不应突出,踏面下方不得透空。楼梯地面应采用防滑材料,所有踏步上的防滑条、警示条等附着物均不应突出踏面。上下楼梯墙面应安装扶杆。

5.1.8.3 内厅、廊应设置休息座椅;老年人居住用房走廊应设置扶杆。

5.1.8.4 老年人居住用房宜设置阳台,开敞式阳台栏杆高度不应低于 1.10 m,且距地面 0.30 m 高度范围内不宜留空,开敞式阳台应做好雨水遮挡及排水措施。

5.1.8.5 严寒及寒冷地区、多风沙地区老年人居住用房宜设封闭阳台。多层或高层建筑及失智老年人居住用房宜采用封闭阳台。

5.1.8.6 医养结合机构辅助设施应利于老年人方便和安全,应具有防碰撞伤害性保护措施和防滑倒措施。

5.1.8.7 老年人居室、活动场所的各种设施设备应安全、稳固、无尖角及尖锐棱边部分。

5.1.8.8 失能、失智老人床位应安置床档;介助老人床位应设置防护垫、安全扶手等。

5.1.8.9 老人居住用房床头、厕所、浴室、公共活动用房、康复与医疗用房应设紧急呼叫装置,呼叫装置高度距地宜为 1.20 m～1.30 m,卫生间呼叫装置高度距地为 0.40 m～0.50 m。

5.1.8.10 老年人健身康复、文化娱乐和休闲活动场所应设置电视监控系统及呼叫报警系统。

5.1.8.11 医养结合机构各出入口、走廊、楼梯间、电梯厅和电梯轿厢等场所应设置安全监控设施。

5.1.9 其他用房

5.1.9.1 养老设施建筑内宜每层设置或集中设置污物间,且污物间应靠近污物运输通道,并应有污物处理及消毒设施。

5.1.9.2 库房设置应符合 GB 50016 要求,物品分类置放,库房不应靠近老年人居住用房。

5.2 康复设施设置要求

5.2.1 多层养老设施宜集中建设康复设备区。

5.2.2 康复设备区应根据养老院规模大小设置器械室间数,每间面积应大于 40 m²,应有窗户直接朝向室外开敞环境,光线充足,通风良好。不应设置在地下室或半地下室。

5.2.3 各种康复健身器材应符合 GB 24436 要求,并做好无伤害化处理,表面圆钝、光滑、无棱角。

5.2.4 应设置手法康复室(手法按摩、功能锻炼),根据养老院规模大小设置康复室间数,每间面积不应小于 20 m²。应有窗户直接朝向室外开敞环境,光线充足,通风良好。

5.2.5 应设置中医治疗室(传统针灸、艾灸、拔罐等),根据养老院规模大小设置治疗室间数,应男女分设,每间不应小于 20 m²,应有窗户直接朝向室外开敞环境,光线充足,通风良好,且应安装排风换气设施。不应设置在地下室或半地下室。

5.2.6 应设置中药浴疗浴足室(传统中药泡浴、浴足),应男女分设,每间不应小于 20 m²。应有窗户直接朝向室外开敞环境,光线充足,通风良好,且应安装排风换气设施。

5.3 医疗设施设置要求

5.3.1 医疗机构建设应符合 GB 51039 要求。

5.3.2 医疗机构设施设备最低标准应符合原国家卫生部[《综合医院分级管理标准(试行)》A3ZDYY-NY-20070924055]要求。

5.3.3 养老院或养护院内自设医务室应符合原国家卫生和计划生育委员会[《养老机构医务室基本标准》(试行)]要求。

5.3.4 养老院或养护院内设护理站应符合原国家卫生和计划生育委员会［《养老机构护理站基本标准》（试行）］要求。

5.3.5 医养结合服务机构医疗机构应设置在养老院（养护院）附近，并设置直通道路。

5.3.6 大型养老院宜自建设等级综合医院或康复医院（二级以上）、中医医院等医疗机构。无自建医疗机构的大型养老院（养护院）应与邻近等级综合医院或康复医院（二级以上）建立依托医院关系。

5.3.7 无自建医院的小型或中型养老院或护理院除应按原国家卫生和计划生育委员会《养老机构医务室基本标准（试行）》（2014）设医务室外，还应与就近医疗机构签订合作协议，委托外部医疗机构提供健康咨询、门诊就医、医生巡诊和双向转诊等医疗服务。

5.4 医疗服务机构与养老服务机构间的链接设施要求

5.4.1 医疗机构与养老机构应实现网络信息化，互联互通，信息共享。

5.4.2 应满足机构和患者家属之间的沟通要求。

5.4.3 医院与养老服务机构（养老院、养护院、日间照护中心和社区）间应建立有线或无线网络会诊平台。

5.4.4 非医养结合机构自建医院（依托医院）应与协作医养结合养老机构（养老院、养护院、日间照护中心和社区）建立有线或无线网络会诊平台。

5.4.5 医养结合机构内自建医院应每周对养老机构定期查房和会诊，指导养老机构医疗活动。

5.4.6 医院应设置专用救护车辆服务于养老服务机构（养老院、养护院、日间照护中心和社区）。

5.4.7 大型医养结合机构自建医院可设置移动式医疗服务车。

参 考 文 献

[1]　《社区老年人日间照料中心建设标准(2010)》国家民政部

[2]　《综合医院分级管理标准(试行)》A3ZDYY-NY-20070924055 国家卫生部

[3]　《康复医院基本标准(试行)》(2012)国家卫生部

[4]　《关于促进健康服务业发展的若干意见》国发[2013]40 号

[5]　《养老机构医务室基本标准(试行)》(2014)国家卫生部

[6]　《养老机构护理站基本标准(试行)》(2014)国家卫生部

[7]　《全国医院信息化建设标准与规范(试行)》(2018)国家卫生健康委员会

[8]　《医疗机构基本标准(试行)》(2018)国家卫生健康委员会

————————————

ICS 03.080
A 20

Social Organization Standard

T/CGSS 005—2019

Basic requirements for infrastructure for service institutions of combination of medical and senior health care

医养结合服务机构设施设置基本要求

（*English Translation*）

Issue date：2019-04-28

Implementation date：2019-04-28

Issued by Chinese Geriatrics Society

Foreword

This standard was drafted in accordance with the rules given in the GB/T 1.1—2009.

This standard was proposed by Department of Integrated Medical and Nursing Management, Department of Standardization Management of Chinese Geriatrics Society.

This standard was prepared by Chinese Geriatrics Society.

This standard was drafted by Promotion Committee of Medical Care Integration of Chinese Geriatrics Society, Chinese PLA General Hospital, National Clinical Research, Center of Geriatrics Disease (Chinese PLA General Hospital), Institute of Architectural Environmental Art Design of China IPPR International Engineering Co., Ltd., Liaoning Zhongzhi Shengjing Hospital of Geriatrics, Qingcheng International Care Center of Chengdu in Sichuan Province, Xinhexin Health and Senior Care Investment Limited Company of Guilin in Guangxi, Kaixuan Elderly Hospital of Linyi in Shandong Province, Health Commission of Shenyang, the Fifth Affiliated Hospital of Zhengzhou University, the Eighth People's Hospital of Chengdu in Sichuan Province, the Third People's Hospital of Gansu Province, the Second People's Hospital of Changzhi in Shanxi Province, Binzhou Medical College of Shandong Province and Home for the Aged Guangzhou.

The main drafters of this standard were Tingshu Yang, Zongyao Long, Shengqiang Jiao, Qun Wang, Feng Lin, Zhijun Sun, Qiang Wu, Lihong Cheng, Changchun Yang, Huiru Hou, Yaogai Li, Weihua Xu, Yafei Zhang, Kaitian Jiang, Pengyuan Zheng, Hailang Huang, Liping Lu, Buqing Wang, Yuling Hao, Lianqi Liu, Liannong Xiao, Shao Chen and Dongke Li.

Introduction

The current population above the age of 60 in China is about 250 million. Population has been aging and the number of empty nesters has been increasing. Thus, the number of elder populations with disabilities has been continuously increasing, potentially resulting in the imbalance between the high demand and limited supply of care services.

The 19th national congress of the Communist Party of China addresses that the health level of a population is an important indicator of the prosperity level of a society and a nation. The government will take proactive measures for population aging issues, create a supportive and respectful environment and adopt policies designed for offering elderly care services, age-friendly service, and engaging medical services with elderly care services and focus on developing healthcare industry for aging population. The Government Work Report published at the Second Session of the Thirteenth National People's Congress of the People's Republic of China, also addresses the focus on developing elderly care services, especially community-based elderly care services, and indicates that we will strive to reform and improve the health policies for engaging medical services with the elderly care services, so that the elderly will enjoy a happy life in their later years.

At present, a variety of care service institutions have developed rapidly and been providing services in China. A new form of care provider that combines medical service and elderly care services has been growing widely across the nation, with various functions such as medical care, elderly care and rehabilitation care. To further develop, manage and regulate such care providing institutions, this standard provides the basic requirements of insfrastructure for service institutions of combination of medical and senior health care.

Basic requirements for infrastructure for service institutions of combination of medical and senior health care

1 Scope

This standard specifies the basic requirements for infrastructure for service institutions that provide combinely medical and senior health care.

This standard is applicable to service institutions that provide combinedly medical and senior health care.

2 Normative references

The following referenced documents are indispensable for the application of this document. For dated references, only the edition cited applies. For undated references, the latest edition of the referenced document (including any amendments) applies.

GB 2894   Safety signs and guideline for the use

GB/T 10001.1   Public information graphical symbols—Part 1: General symbols

GB 18466   Discharge standard of water pollutants for medical organization

GB/T 18883   Indoor air quality standard

GB 24436   Rehabilitation training instrument— General safety requirements

GB 50011   Code for seismic design of buildings

GB 50016   Code for fire protection design of buildings

GB 50019   Design code for heating ventilation and air conditioning of industrial buildings

GB 50034   Standard for lighting design of buildings

GB 50763　Code for accessibility design

GB 51039　Code for design of general hospitals

JGJ 450　Standard for architectural design of elderly care service facilities

3　Terms and definitions

For the purposes of this document, the terms and definitions given in JGJ 450 and the following apply.

3.1
service institutions of combination of medical and senior health care

an institution with both medical and elderly care qualifications and capabilities to provide combinedly medical and elderly care services as well as health management services

3.2
senior nursing home
geriatric nursing home

an institution provides comprehensive services such as daily care, medical care and rehabilitation care as well as cultural and recreational activities for the elderly

3.3
day care center for the aged

an institution provides comprehensive services such as daily care, meals, basic nursing, physical therapy and rehabilitation, cultural and recreational activities, as well as transportation and other assistance for the dependent elderly

3.4
nursing unit

a relatively independent facility designed to provide nursing care and maintain care quality

3.5
nursing bed

a facility with beds adapted to the needs of the elderly with physical and mental disabilities

4 General principles

4.1 Service institutions of combination of medical and senior health care shall adhere to the principles of being customer-centric, scientific, reasonable and applicable. Facilities shall meet the needs of the elderly for basic daily care, nursing rehabilitation, health care, pshychological comfort and hospice care.

4.2 Service institutions combination of medical and senior health care shall provide elderly care services based on the physiological characteristics of the elderly, understand the environmental needs of the elderly,and strive to provide an adaptable, comfortable, safe and reliable environment for them.

4.3 Service institutions combination of medical and senior health care shall emphasize the advantage of combining proper medical and elderly care services, and understand the specials needs for the elderly with common diseases and chronic medical conditions. It is crucial to meet the elderly's medical demand of treatments for common diseases and chronic diseases. The design of medical specialty facility and care services shall facilitate the treatment of senile deseases and rehabilitation of chronic conditions and be beneficial to the elderly's physical and mental health.

5 Basic requirements

5.1 Requirements of infrastrure for elderly care service

5.1.1 Site selection and facility layout

5.1.1.1 Site selection and layout of care service institutions shall be scientific and reasonable. It shall meet the requirements of JGJ 450.

5.1.1.2 Site selection shall avoid locations near wind gaps, river, and moutains with mudflow risks and locations of any other potential geological safety hazards.

5.1.1.3 It is recommended to be adjacent to public landscapes and recreational places, such as parks, cultural centers, playgrounds in the city and have access to public service facilities nearby.

5.1.1.4 There shall be both indoor and outdoor space reserved for recreational, fitness and entertainment activities etc. for the elderly. The average area per person shall not be less than 1.20 m^2.

5.1.1.5 Area space for landscaping and gardening shall be reserved within service facilities. Trees, shrubs and flowers as well as lawns are recommended.

5.1.1.6 Decorative fountains are recommended for facility design. The depth of fountains should not exceed 0. 6 m. Safety signs and security measures are required.

5. 1. 1. 7 Public toilets, benches, lighting system, awnings and sun/rain shades shall be available for use in the public areas and activity places.

5. 1. 1. 8 The design of barrier-free facilities in public areas and activity places shall meet the requirements of GB 50763.

5. 1. 1. 9 Barbershops, stores, banks, post offices, insurance agents and other convenience services shall be included in the design of any large-size nursing facilities.

5. 1. 1. 10 Public parking lots shall be reserved in the newly-constructed nursing facilities, and the ratio of parking spots to nursing beds shall be 0. 1/1.

5. 1. 1. 11 Signs and graphic symbols shall be obvious in public areas, and the design and use of signs shall meet the requirements of GB/T 10001. 1 and GB 2894.

5. 1. 2 Requirements of facility construction

5. 1. 2. 1 The architectural design of medical and nursing institutions shall meet the requirements of JGJ 450.

5. 1. 2. 2 Seismic design of any residential buildings shall meet the requirements of GB 50011.

5. 1. 2. 3 The design of fire protection systems of residential buildings shall meet the requirements of GB 50016.

5. 1. 2. 4 The minimum ceiling height of residential space for the elderly should not be less than 2. 60 m. There shall be sufficient indoor day light exposure, and the duration of sunshine exposure should not be less than 2 h during winter time. Effective ventilation is necessary.

5. 1. 2. 5 The width of bedroom doors shall not be less than 1. 10 m for the elderly. The width of bathroom doors shall not be less than 0. 90 m. The width of residential hallways and corridors shall not be less than 2. 10 m. The width of hallways and corridors in the public areas is recommended to be 2. 40 m and shall not be less than 2. 10 m.

5. 1. 2. 6 Elderly care housing buildings should bemainly low-rise and multi-layer. Buildings of more than two stories shall be equipped with multiple elevators, including accessible elevators. Elevators shall be able to acommendate medical beds, flatbeds and stretcher beds. Buildings with more than two stories shall be equipped with at least one elevator per every 100 to 120 nuring beds.

5. 1. 2. 7 It is recommended to reserve designated parking space for ambulances, shuttles and grocery delivery vehicles. Designated storage spaces for flatcars, stretchers, wheelchairs and other vehicles for transportation are required.

5.1.2.8 The exit of garage should be connected directly to the main traffic to provide easy access for ambulances and other vehicles used for elderly's daily transportation.

5.1.3 Requirements of indoor construction

5.1.3.1 Water supply and drainage system

5.1.3.1.1 Hot water supply system of elderly care facilities shall meet the requirements of GB 50019. Hot water shall be supplied 24 hours in a whole day. The water temperature at the distribution point should be 40 ℃~50 ℃. It shall be equipped with temperature control and pressure stabilization devices.

5.1.3.1.2 Drainage system shall be always functional. The contamination level of water discharge from medical facilities shall meet the requirements of GB 18466. There shall be independent water pipes and discharge shall be centralized to the unified treatment tank for disinfection treatment.

5.1.3.2 Heating, ventilation and air conditioning systems

5.1.3.2.1 Elerly care service institutions in severe cold and cold areas shall equip with central heating systems. It is recommended to use low-temperature hot water floor radiant heating systems. Institutions in areas with hot summer and cold winter shall have heating facilities.

5.1.3.2.2 Indoor temperature level of care facilities shall meet the requirements of GB 50019. The temperature with heating shall not be lower than 22 ℃ in winter, and the temperature shall not be higher than 28 ℃ in summer.

5.1.3.2.3 Air quality in care facilities shall meet the requirements of GB/T 18883. Public kitchens, private and public bathrooms shall be equipped with ventilation system and installed with mechanical exhaust fans. The mechanical exhaust fan system shall have the backflow preventers.

5.1.3.2.4 Air conditioning system in care facilities shall be able to accomendate temperature control for each individual room.

5.1.3.2.5 Vibration and noise reduction measures shall be installed for any noise-generating equipment such as water pumps and fans used in the buildings of care facilities.

5.1.3.3 Electrical lighting system

5.1.3.3.1 The lighting of living space, activity areas and any auxiliary spaces in care facilities shall meet the requirements of GB 50034. It is recommended to choose energy-saving and warm tone lights. The color rendering index of the lighting source should be more than 80, and the glare index should be less than 19.

5.1.3.3.2 Emergency lights shall be installed in residential rooms and public activity spaces in care facilities. It is recommended to be automatically controlled.

5.1.3.3.3 The lighting of residential rooms, bathrooms and corridors and hallways shall meet the requirements of JGJ 450. It is recommended to install embedded footlights. Multiway switching light control should be installed for ceiling lights of bedrooms and long corridors.

5.1.3.3.4 The lighting control switch in care facilities shall meet the requirements of JGJ 450. Light switches with wider boards are recommended.

5.1.3.3.5 Illumination lights shall be installed in corridors, staircases, balconies and elevator halls in the facilities. Emergency lights shall also be installed in corridors and staircases. Sound and light control system is recommended for emergency lights.

5.1.3.3.6 Power outlets installed in the facilities shall meet the requirements of JGJ 450. When the power outlets are installed lower than 1.8 m above the ground, safety power outlets shall be used.

5.1.3.3.7 TV, telephone and internet cables shall be installed in residential rooms, public activity areas and public restaurants of care facilities, etc.

5.1.3.3.8 The power supply of care facilities shall be safe and reliable. Special electrical wire should be used for electricity distribution, and the design of power supply and distribution system shall be concise and clear. In addition, the power supply and distribution wires shall be hidden.

5.1.4 Requirements of indoor living facility

5.1.4.1 Elderly care institutions shall be divided into one or more nursing units according to their sizes. Each floor of high-rise buildings should be defined as a nursing unit. The number of total beds recommended for each nursing unit is 50~100, and the number of total beds for nursing home for the elderly only shall not be more than 50.

5.1.4.2 Housing arrangement shall meet the requirements of JGJ 450. Based on the number of beds there are one-bed rooms, two-beds rooms and multiple-beds rooms. The area of a one-bed room shall not be less than 10 m^2, and the area of a two-beds room shall not be less than 16 m^2. The area of a multiple-beds room shall be based on the number of beds. The average net floor area per bed shall not be less than 6 m^2.

5.1.4.3 Each room in nursing home shall have no more than 4 regular beds or no more than 6 nursing beds. The gap space between two beds shall not be less than 0.80 m. The distance between the bed and day lighting exterior wall shall not be less than 0.60 m. The distance between aisle bed and wall shall not be less than 1. 05 m.

5. 1. 4. 4   It is recommended that the number of beds in each bedroom varies from 2 to 4 and shall be no more than 4.

5. 1. 4. 5   The construction design of community day care centers for the elderly shall meet the requirements of *Construction standards of community daycare centers for the elderly (2010)* by the Ministry of Civil Affairs of the People's Republic of China. The capacity number of the elderly in care suggested in each elderly lounge is 4~8.

5. 1. 4. 6   There shall be enough number of bedside cabinets and storage bureaus based on the number of beds in each room. The storage bureaus shall have easy access for the elderly. They shall not be taller than 1. 60 m used for the elderly in wheelchairs.

5. 1. 4. 7   In addition to the space for beds, there should be enough space for wheelchairs, flat cars and hospital beds in each care room of a nursing center. There shall be enough bedside space to accomendate any nursing and first aid activities.

5. 1. 4. 8   There shall be private bathrooms including toilets, washing sinks and shower rooms in each nursing care room. Sitting toilet and shower shall be in the bathrooms. Safety handrails shall be installed for the toilet, washing sink and shower rooms.

5. 1. 4. 9   The space for auxiliary facilities shall be considered in the layout of bathroom design for the elderly with disabilities.

5. 1. 5   Requirements of dining room facility

5. 1. 5. 1   The usable area of public dining room shall meet the requirements of JGJ 450.

5. 1. 5. 2   It is recommended to have public dining rooms for medical care and nursing care areas separately. One public dining room should be available for each care unit. A dining room shall not serve more than 50 people, and a feeding bed shall not be smaller than 0. 93 m^2.

5. 1. 5. 3   Small public dining rooms and food prep rooms shall be available on each floor of high-rise nursing care buildings.

5. 1. 5. 4   Public dining rooms shall use mobile yet stury and stable single chairs.

5. 1. 5. 5   The layout of public dining room shall reserve enough space to acommedate food serving carts and areas for nursing staff to prepare food and help feed the elderly. Barrier-free counter design is recommended when food is ordered and delivered from the counter.

5. 1. 5. 6   Food prep rooms may be set up close to the public dining areas. A food prep room shall not

be no less than 10 m². A food prep room is designed for the caregivers to distribute, heat and cut food for the incapable elderly.

5.1.5.7 Kitchens shall not be built adjacent to the living space of the elderly. The kitchen exhaust emission system shall be directed towards open areas, and fume emission system shall be controlled to avoid contaminating living areas.

5.1.6 Requirements of recreational room facilities

5.1.6.1 Large high-rise care facilities shall have public recreational and activity area on each floor. Area per capita shall not be less than 1.20 m², and shall have sufficient lighting, and ventilation and be appropriate for recreational activities.

5.1.6.2 Each nursing unit in care facilities shall have a recreational room for reading newspapers, playing chess and card games. The room area shall not be less than 20 m², and the room shall have sufficient sunlight and good ventilation.

5.1.6.3 Each nursing unit shall have a designated family room (may be used as a psychological consulting room) with an area of no less than 12 m². Simple furniture such as a sofa and a tea table is recommended for visitors and the elderly's use. The family room shall have enough sunlight and good ventilation.

5.1.6.4 Fitness centers and gyms with appropriate exercise equipment are recommended.

5.1.7 Requirements of information technology system

5.1.7.1 Service institutions of combination of medical and senior health care shall be able to set up internet wire and outlet to deploy information technology systems for information management, network services and video transmission purposes.

5.1.7.2 The deployment of hospital information technology systems shall follow the requirements of *National standards and norms for hospital information technology construction* (*trial*)(*2018*) by National Health Commission.

5.1.7.3 Service institutions of combination of medical and senior health care shall have internet platform for remote medical consultation.

5.1.7.4 Residential rooms of the elderly shall be equipped with cable TV, telephone and indoor mobile communication devices.

5.1.8 Special safety requirements

5.1.8.1 The design of barrier-free channel of entrances and exits, passageways, corridors and indoor entrances and exits in the medical and nursing homes shall meet the requirements of GB 50763.

5.1.8.2   The stair nosing shall not have any overhang, and the stair tread shall not use any transparent material. All stairs shall use slippery-resistant material. Any anti-slip strips of stairs, warning signs and other stair attachments shall not over hang to cause any trip and fall risks. Safety handrails shall be installed for all staircases.

5.1.8.3   Resting chairs and benches shall be provided inside medical and nursing homes and in the hallways. Safety handrails shall be installed in the hallways of the elderly residential buildings.

5.1.8.4   It is recommended to have balconies for the elderly's living rooms. The height of safety handrails of any open balcony shall not be lower than 1.10 m. The buttom side of the handrails shall not be taller than 0.30 m above the ground. Awnings and gutters shall be installed for open balconies.

5.1.8.5   It is recommended to chose closed balconies for the elderly residents in cold, windy and sandy areas. Multi-story or high-rise buildings and facilities for the elderly with mental disabilities should construct closed balconies.

5.1.8.6   Any auxiliary facilities used in service institutions of combination of medical and senior health care shall be convenient and safe for the elderly to use. Protective measures such as collision-resistant devices and anti-slippery measures shall be taken.

5.1.8.7   Equipments and devices used in living rooms and activity places for the elderly shall be safe, stable and free from sharp objects and sharp edges.

5.1.8.8   Protective bedrails shall be installed for the elderly with physical or mental disabilities. Safety devices such as cushion pads and handrails shall be installed for the elderly who need aid devices.

5.1.8.9   Emergency call devices shall be installed at bedsides, toilets, bathrooms, public activity rooms, rehabilitation and medical rooms for the elderly. The call devices should be installed at the height of 1.20 m~1.30 m above the ground. The call devices used in bathrooms should be installed at the height of 0.40 m~0.50 m above the ground.

5.1.8.10   Cable camera system and emergency call system shall be installed at rehabilitation, entertainment and recreational activity areas for the elderly.

5.1.8.11   Safety survelliance system shall be installed at entrances, hallways, staircases and elevators at the facilities that provide medical and nursing care services.

5.1.9 Other uses of occupancy

5.1.9.1 Trash and disposal rooms should be available on each floor or at a centralized area of the building. The trash and disposal rooms shall be connected to the disposal transportation channel and equipped with disinfection treatment facilities.

5.1.9.2 The storage rooms shall meet the requirements of GB 50016. Storage rooms shall be used by categories. The storage rooms shall not be adjacent to the elderly's bedrooms.

5.2 Requirements of rehabilitation facilities

5.2.1 There should be a central rehabilitation area in any multi-story buildings of nursing care facilities.

5.2.2 The number of equipment rooms for rehabilitation use depends on the size of a nursing home. Each equipment room shall have an area more than 40 m^2 and with windows facing directly the outside open air as well as sufficient sunlight and good ventilation. The rehabilitation areas shall not be in the basement or semi-basement.

5.2.3 Any fitness equipment used for rehabilitation purpose shall meet the requirements of GB 24436. All equipments shall be made of harmless material, with a dull, smooth surface and without edges or corners.

5.2.4 Designated areas for manual rehabilitation including manual massage and functional exercise shall be provided. The number of physical therapy rooms depends on the size of the nursing home. Each physical therapy room shall not be less than 20 m^2 and with windows facing directly the outside open air as well as sufficient sunlight and good ventilation.

5.2.5 Treatment rooms used for traditional Chinese medicine treatment (traditional acupuncture, moxibustion, cupping, etc.) shall be provided. The number of treatment rooms depends on the size of the nursing home, and shall be provided separately for men and women. Each treatment room shall be no less than 20 m^2 and with windows facing directly the outside open air as well as sufficient sunlight and good ventilation. The treatment rooms shall not be in basement or semi-basement.

5.2.6 Bathing rooms used for medicated bath and foot bathing therapy (traditional Chinese medicine bath and foot bath) shall be provided separately for men and women. The area of each bathing room shall not be less than 20 m^2 and with windows facing directly the outside open air as well as sufficient light and good ventilation. Exhaust ventilation system shall be installed.

5.3 Requirements of medical facility

5.3.1 The construction of medical institutions shall meet the requirements of GB 51039.

5.3.2　The minimum standards of facilities and equipments in medical institutions shall meet the requirements of *Classification management standards of comprehensive hospital*（*trial*）A3ZDYY-NY-20070924055 issued by the former National Ministry of Health.

5.3.3　Self-managed medical clinics of nursing homes or elderly care service institutions shall meet the requirements of *Basic standards of infirmary in ederly care institutions*（*trial*），issued by the former National Health and Family Planning Commission.

5.3.4　Nursing stations of nursing homes and elderly care service institutions shall meet the requirements of *Basic standards of nursing stations in elderly care institutions*（*trial*），issued by the former National Health and Family Planning Commission.

5.3.5　Service institutions of combination of mdical and senior health care shall be located near nursing homes（elderly service homes）and set up direct passages.

5.3.6　Large-sized nursing homes should be encouraged to establish medical institutions such as integrated comprehensive hospitals，rehabilitation hospitals（above grade 2）and traditional Chinese medicine hospitals，etc. The large-sized nursing homes without self-managed medical institutions shall establish collaborative relationships with graded integrated hospitals or rehabilitation hospitals（above grade 2）.

5.3.7　Small or medium-sized care service institutions or nursing homes without self-built hospitals shall not only develop medical facilities according to the *Basic Standards of Nursing Rooms for the Elderly*（*Trial*）issued by the former National Health and Family Planning Commission，but also establish cooperation agreements with nearby medical institutions to entrust external medical institutions to provide healthcare consultation，outpatient treatment，doctor's patro，two-way referral and other medical services.

5.4　Relationship between medical service institutions and care service institutions

5.4.1　Medical service institutions and care service institutions shall realize network informatization，interconnection and information sharing.

5.4.2　Communication requirements between the institutions and the patient's family shall be met.

5.4.3　Wired or wireless internet network platforms for medical consultation shall be established between the hospitals and nursing institutions（nursing institutions，elderly care service institutions，day care centers and communities）.

5.4.4　Wired or wireless internet network platforms for medical consultation shall be established between self-built hospitals in non-medical and nursing institutions（dependent on the hospitals）and collaborative medical and nursing care institutions for the elderly（care homes，maintenance homes，day care centers and communities）.

5.4.5 Self-built hospitals in medical care and nursing institutions shall make weekly medical visits and consultations at the elderly care service institutions to provide guidance of medical activities of the elderly care institutions.

5.4.6 Hospitals shall reserve designated ambulances to serve elderly care service institutions（care homes，nursing homes，day care centers and communities）.

5.4.7 Mobile medical service vehicles may be available in self-built hospitals of large-scale medical and nursing institutions.

Bibliography

[1] Construction standards for community day care centers for the elderly (2010), Ministry of Civil Affairs of the People's Republic of China

[2] A3ZDYY-NY-20070924055, Classification and management standards of comphrehensive hospitals (trial), National Ministry of Health

[3] Basic standards of rehabilitation hospitals (trial)(2012), National Ministry of Health

[4] Several opinions on promoting the development of health service industry, National Development and Reform Commission [2013]No. 40

[5] Basic standards of infirmary in ederly care institutions (trial) (2014), National Ministry of Health

[6] Basic standards of nursing stations in elderly care institutions (trial)(2014), National Ministry of Health

[7] National standards and norms for hospital information technology construction (trial)(2018) , National Health Commission

[8] Basic standards for medical institutions (trial) (2018),National Health Commission

---

ICS 03.080.99

A 20

团 体 标 准

T/CGSS 006—2019

医养结合服务机构等级评定规范

Grade assessment specification for service institutions of
combination of medical and senior health care

2019-04-28 发布

2019-04-28 实施

中国老年医学学会 发 布

前　言

本标准按照 GB/T 1.1—2009 给出的规则起草。

本标准由中国老年医学学会医养结合管理部和标准化管理部提出。

本标准由中国老年医学学会归口。

本标准起草单位：中国老年医学学会医养结合促进委员会、解放军总医院、国家老年疾病临床研究中心（解放军总医院）、中国中元国际工程有限公司建筑环境艺术设计研究院、辽宁省沈阳中置盛京老年医院、四川省成都青城国际颐养中心、广西壮族自治区桂林信和信健康养老产业投资有限公司、山东省临沂市凯旋老年医院、沈阳市卫生健康委员会、郑州大学第五附属医院、四川省成都市第八人民医院、甘肃省第三人民医院、山西省长治市第二人民医院、山东省滨州医学院、广州市老人院。

本标准主要起草人：杨庭树、龙宗耀、焦胜强、王群、林峰、孙志军、武强、程丽红、杨长春、侯惠如、李瑶盖、徐卫华、章亚非、姜开田、郑鹏远、黄海浪、鲁丽萍、王补青、郝玉玲、刘联琦、肖联农、陈芍、李东科。

引　言

目前我国 60 岁以上人口约达 2.5 亿,社会老龄化、"空巢化"程度不断加深,失能、半失能老年人不断增多,养老服务供需矛盾突出。

党的十九大指出,人民健康是民族昌盛和国家富强的重要标志。要积极应对人口老龄化,构建养老、孝老、敬老政策体系和社会环境,推动医养结合,加快老龄事业和产业发展。十三届人大二次会议政府工作报告指出,要大力发展养老特别是社区养老服务业,改革完善医养结合政策,使老年人拥有幸福的晚年。

目前,我国多种多样的养老服务机构发展迅速,以医疗资源和养老资源有机协同为一体的新型医疗护理、养老照护、康复养生型的养老服务也在全国各地广泛开展。为引领、促进和规范医养结合服务机构的发展,特制定医养结合服务机构等级评定规范。

医养结合服务机构等级评定规范

1 范围

本标准规定了医养结合服务机构等级划分与标识、申请等级评定应具备的基本要求与条件、等级评定组织与管理。

本标准适用于医养结合服务机构等级划分与评定。

2 规范性引用文件

下列文件对于本文件的应用是必不可少的。凡是注日期的引用文件，仅注日期的版本适用于本文件。凡是不注日期的引用文件，其最新版本（包括所有的修改单）适用于本文件。

GB/T 29353 养老机构基本规范

GB/T 35796 养老机构服务质量基本规范

GB/T 37276 养老机构等级划分与评定

MZ/T 039 老年人能力评估

JGJ 450 老年人照料设施建筑设计标准

T/CGSS 001 老年照护师规范

T/CGSS 005 医养结合服务机构设施设置基本要求

3 术语和定义

GB/T 37276、T/CGSS 005 界定的以及下列术语和定义适用于本文件。

3.1

医养结合服务机构 service institutions of combination of medical and senior health care

具有医疗、养老两方面的资质和/或能力并能提供医疗、养老服务和健康管理相结合的机构。

3.2

等级 grade

在综合考评养老机构的环境、设施设备、运营管理和服务的基础上所做的分级。

3.3

机构入住率 occupancy rate

入住老年人总数与养老机构内总床位数的比率（％）。

3.4

医疗服务 medical care services

为养老机构老年人提供基本医疗、预防、保健、康复和健康管理的活动。

3.5

护理服务 nursing services

执业护士按照护理常规诊断和处置老年人现存的或潜在的健康问题及指导护理员、照护士（师）完成对老年人的生活照料、基础护理和心理护理活动。

4 总则

4.1 等级评定工作应做到全面客观、质量为重、注重实效、公正公平,确保评定结论的公信力。

4.2 等级评定的重点是基本要求和基本条件。基本要求作为等级评定的必要条件,基本条件则是等级评定确定等级的必要条件。

4.3 等级评定的重要指标是服务设施和服务内容应与服务区域、服务人群、服务需求相适应,应重点关注老年人养老照护、健康保障、康复养生,应注重服务内容和服务质量。

5 等级分类

5.1 医养结合服务机构规模分类

5.1.1 医院等级规模应按原国家卫生部《综合医院分级管理标准(试行)》A3ZDYY-NY-20070924055规定执行。

5.1.2 养老服务机构规模分为大、中、小3个类型(见表1)。

表 1 养老服务机构床位数规模(张)

机构类型	床位规模/张		
	大型	中型	小型
养老院	≥501	151~500	≤150
老年养护院	≥301	101~300	≤100
社区日间老年照护中心	≥101	51~100	≤50

5.2 医养结合服务机构等级分类

5.2.1 等级划分

按医养结合服务机构建设规模和服务能力分为5个等级,从低到高依次为一级、二级、三级、四级和五级医养结合服务机构。级数越高,表示医养结合服务机构建设规模、设施设备、环境布局、运营管理、服务内容和服务质量等方面更强。

5.2.2 等级标识

等级标识由五角星图案构成。一颗五角星表示为一级、两颗五角星表示为二级、三颗五角星表示为三级、四颗五角星表示为四级、五颗五角星表示为五级。

示例:五级医养结合服务机构标识示意图见图1。

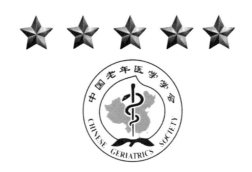

中 国 老 年 医 学 学 会 制

图 1 等级标识

6 申请等级评定的基本要求和基本条件

6.1 申请等级评定的基本要求

6.1.1 医养结合服务机构养老设施设备应符合 GB/T 29353 和 T/CGSS 005 的要求。

6.1.2 医养结合服务机构应具备以下有效执业证明：

　　a) 养老机构设置应具备"社会福利机构设置批准证书"、有效的"营业执照"或"事业单位法人证书"或"民办非企业单位登记证书"；医疗机构设置应具备"医疗机构执业许可证"；

　　b) 房产证明或租赁协议；消防审验合格证明或消防备案证明；

　　c) 餐饮服务机构应具备食品卫生经营许可证；

　　d) 特种设备，应具备相应的特种设备使用登记证，包括但不限于电梯、锅炉使用登记证等。

6.1.3 医养结合服务机构人员资质要求：

　　a) 医生应持有"医师资格证书"和"医师执业证书"；护士应持有"护士执业证书"；其他专业人员应持有相适应的专业资格证书及执业证书。老年照护师和/或养老护理员应符合国家相关规定和 T/CGSS 001 要求或经执业技能培训合格后上岗。

　　b) 所有工作人员均应持有健康证明。

6.1.4 建立完善的基本管理制度，应符合 GB/T 35796 要求，还应包括但不限于：

　　a) 办公管理制度；

　　b) 出入院管理及随访制度；

　　c) 服务管理及质量控制制度；

　　d) 医师查房会诊制度；

　　e) 医疗操作查对制度；

　　f) 健康管理及病历书写制度；

　　g) 应急值班制度；

　　h) 医-养机构双向转诊及"绿色通道制度"；

　　i) 信息管理制度；

　　j) 人力资源管理制度；

　　k) 财务管理及专项资金管理制度；

　　l) 后勤管理制度；

　　m) 安全管理制度，包括但不限于食品安全管理制度、设施设备安全管理制度；

　　n) 医疗废弃物管理制度。

6.1.5　医养结合服务机构等级评定内容和分值的基本要求见表 A.1。

6.2　申请等级评审应具备的基本条件

6.2.1　一级医养结合服务机构

6.2.1.1　符合 5.1.1 医养服务机构建设规模"小型"标准。

6.2.1.2　应设置医务室和护理站。且应符合原国家卫生和计划生育委员会《养老机构医务室基本标准（试行）》(2014)和《养老机构护理站基本标准（试行）》(2014)要求。

6.2.1.3　运营管理应符合 6.1 要求。

6.2.1.4　护理人员配置应符合 GB/T 35796 和 GB/T 37276 的要求,每个养护单元至少配置 1 名具有主管护师以上专业职务任职资格的护士和 1 名护士长。

6.2.1.5　持有老年照护师和/或养老护理员初级及以上证书或者经培训达到初级养老护理员标准的人员比例不低于 50%。

6.2.1.6　入住率应符合 GB/T 37276 要求,其中失能失智老年人入住比例应不低于 30%。

6.2.1.7　服务项目除按 GB/T 29353 要求执行外,还应包括出入院服务、老年人能力评估、一般生活照料服务、医疗护理服务、年度查体服务、心理咨询服务、膳食服务、清洁卫生服务、洗涤服务和理发服务等。

6.2.1.8　服务质量应符合 GB/T 35796 要求。

6.2.1.9　应建立网络信息化服务系统,包括但不限于办公网络化、入住老人健康管理网络化及老人出院随访网络化。

6.2.1.10　一年内无责任事故发生、服务质量满意度＞85%并有提升改进措施。

6.2.1.11　等级评定内容和分值的基本条件见表 A.2。

6.2.2　二级医养结合服务机构

6.2.2.1　首先应满足本规范 6.2.1 要求。

6.2.2.2　在符合 5.1.1 医养结合服务机构建设规模"小型"标准的基础上,还应有超市、邮寄、理发等综合服务设施。

6.2.2.3　养老护理人员与入住老年人比例应符合 GB/T 37276 二级养老机构要求。

6.2.2.4　持有养老护理员初级及以上证书或者经培训达到初级养老护理员标准的人员比例不低于 60%。

6.2.2.5　入住率应符合 GB/T 37276 二级养老机构要求,其中失能失智老年人入住比例不应低于 30%。

6.2.2.6　服务项目除包含本规范 6.2.1.7 要求外,还应有安宁疗护服务、心理/精神支持服务、营养评价服务、文化娱乐服务、通信交通服务、邮寄代购服务等。

6.2.2.7　网络信息化服务除符合 6.2.1.9 要求外,应增加与医养结合机构内医疗机构专家咨询的视频网络化会诊系统。

6.2.2.8　一年内无责任事故,服务质量满意度＞90%并有提升改进措施。

6.2.2.9　等级评定内容和分值的基本条件见表 A.3。

6.2.3　三级医养结合服务机构

6.2.3.1　首先应满足本规范 6.2.2 要求。

6.2.3.2　在符合 5.1.1 医养服务机构建设规模"中型"标准的基础上,还应有体育活动室、娱乐室、美容室等综合服务设施,住房内应配备电冰箱、彩色电视机等。

6.2.3.3 有自建等级综合或康复医院(二级以上),或与邻近二级以上综合(康复)医院建立有共享医疗资源协议,并建立互通转诊及重危急症"绿色通道"。

6.2.3.4 每个养护单元应设置医疗处置室和护士站。

6.2.3.5 养老院和老年养护院应设置安宁疗护室,安宁疗护室宜靠近医务室且相对独立,其对外通道不应与养老居住设施建筑入口合用。

6.2.3.6 养老护理人员与入住老年人比例应符合 GB/T 37276 三级养老机构要求。

6.2.3.7 医护人员配置应按原国家卫生部《护理院基本标准(2011 版)》执行。

6.2.3.8 持有老年照护师和/或养老护理员初级及以上证书或者经培训达到初级养老护理员标准的人员比例不低于70%。

6.2.3.9 入住率应符合 GB/T 37276 三级养老机构要求,其中失能失智老年人入住比例不应低于30%。

6.2.3.10 服务项目除包括 6.2.2.6 要求外,还应有舒缓疗护、中医养生、保健服务、体育、文化、娱乐、旅游服务等。

6.2.3.11 养老机构网络信息化服务除符合本规范 6.2.2.7 要求外,还应与本市或本地区主要医疗机构建立密切联系,设置临床医疗指导、疑难病症会诊及急危重症处置"绿色通道"。

6.2.3.12 至少有 1 名社会工作者指导开展社会工作服务。

6.2.3.13 一年内无责任事故发生、服务质量满意度应>95%并有提升改进措施。

6.2.3.14 等级评定内容和分值的基本条件见表 A.4。

6.2.4 四级医养结合服务机构

6.2.4.1 首先应符合本规范 6.2.3 要求。

6.2.4.2 符合 5.1.1 医养结合服务机构建设规模"大型"标准。机构内设备齐全、现代化程度高,综合服务设施完善、服务质量优良,室内环境温馨舒适、室外环境优美。

6.2.4.3 医疗设施应符合 6.2.3.3 要求,应建立与本地区或国内权威医院的技术协作关系,可通过技术交流、人才培训不断提升自身的医疗服务能力。

6.2.4.4 养老护理人员与入住老年人比例应符合 GB/T 37276 四级养老机构要求。

6.2.4.5 持有养老护理员初级及以上证书或者经培训达到初级养老护理员标准的人员比例不低于80%。

6.2.4.6 入住率应符合 GB/T 37276 四级养老机构要求,其中失能失智老年人入住比例不应低于30%。

6.2.4.7 每个养护单元应设置医疗处置室和护士站。

6.2.4.8 服务项目除符合本规范 6.2.3.10 要求外,还应有老年大学、家庭签约服务等。

6.2.4.9 网络信息化服务除符合规范 6.2.3.11 要求外,应与本地区或外地权威医院建立视频网络会诊系统,负责疑难病例会诊、急危重症抢救和手术指导等。

6.2.4.10 至少有 1 名～2 名社会工作者指导开展社会工作服务。

6.2.4.11 一年内无责任事故、服务质量满意度>95%并有提升改进措施。

6.2.4.12 等级评定内容和分值的基本条件见表 A.5。

6.2.5 五级医养结合服务机构

6.2.5.1 首先应符合本规范 6.2.4 要求。

6.2.5.2 符合 5.1.1 医养服务机构建设规模"大型"标准。驻地生态环境优美、设施更加完善、设备更加现代化、服务项目齐全、服务质量高。同时应设有社交、旅游、娱乐、购物、休闲、文化、艺术、养生和健体等活动场所。

6.2.5.3 养老护理人员与入住老年人比例应符合 GB/T 37276 五级养老机构要求。

6.2.5.4 入住率应符合 GB/T 37276 五级养老机构要求,其中失能失智老年人入住率不应低于 30%。

6.2.5.5 服务项目除符合本规范 6.2.4.8 要求外,还应有:种植养植服务、艺术教育服务、社会参与服务、金融与理财服务和法律援助服务等。

6.2.5.6 网络信息化服务除符合本规范 6.2.4.9 要求外,还应建立与国内知名医疗机构的视频网络会诊系统。

6.2.5.7 至少有 2 名社会工作者指导开展社会工作服务。

6.2.5.8 等级评定内容和分值的基本条件见表 A.6。

7 等级评定的组织与管理

7.1 评定委员会组成与职责

中国老年医学学会设立医养结合服务机构等级评定委员会(以下简称:等级评定委员会),并统筹协调全国医养结合服务机构等级评定工作。

7.2 等级评定流程和方法

7.2.1 流程

医养结合服务机构等级评定流程见图 2。

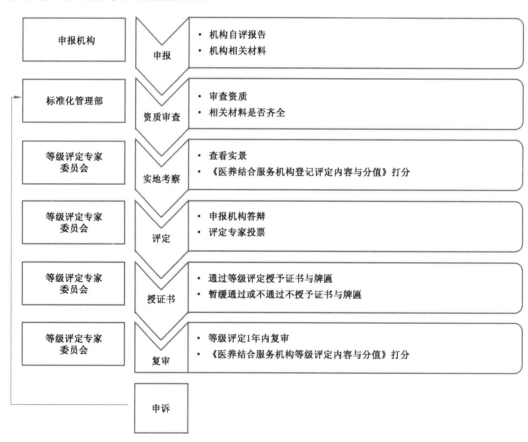

图 2 医养结合服务机构等级评定流程图

7.2.2 方法

7.2.2.1 申报

医养结合服务机构自愿向中国老年医学学会标准化管理部提出申请,并提交自评报告及相关材料。申报材料包括:

    a) 医养结合服务机构养老单位(养老院、养护院、社区日间照护中心)的"社会福利机构设置批准证书""社会福利机构执业证书"及养老机构资质证明;

    b) 医养结合服务机构自建医疗单位(综合医院、康复医院或专科医院、医务室/门诊部)"医疗机构执业许可证"及医院资质证明;

    c) 医养结合服务机构与依托医疗单位的医疗协作协议书,同时出示协作医疗单位"医疗机构执业许可证"及医院资质证明;

    d) 申报单位自评报告,应包括如下内容:

        1) 医养结合服务机构规模,明确申请拟评定等级级别;

        2) 机构内养老、康复、医疗设施设备;

        3) 机构内医疗、医技、护理、照护、后勤及管理人才队伍建设;

        4) 机构试运营情况,重点包括社会和经济效益、质量评估、社会满意度和改进发展措施;

    e) 医养结合服务机构在申报等级评定过程中,发现有下列情况即取消申报等级评定资格:

        1) 存在重大违法、违纪及违规行为;

        2) 违反评定纪律,采取不规范行为影响评定专家的公正公平性,干扰评定专家工作;

        3) 提供虚假评定资料,有伪造档案资料等弄虚作假行为;

        4) 存在医德医风、医疗质量和医疗安全等方面的重大缺陷。

7.2.2.2 资质审查

中国老年医学学会标准化管理部在收到申报材料后的 20 个工作日内对申报单位的申报材料进行资质审查,包括:

    a) 申报单位医疗和养老机构运营资质必须符合国家规定并附有文件(复印件);

    b) 申报单位应符合本规范 7.2.2.1 全部申报条件;

    c) 资质审查结论:通过、补充材料后再审和退回。

7.2.2.3 实地考察

    a) 由评定委员会组织实地考察专家组 5 人以上专家进行实地考察。

    b) 实地考察专家组按"医养结合服务机构等级评定内容及分值"(见附录 A)逐项打分。

    c) 实地考察专家组将申报单位"医养结合服务机构等级评定内容及分值"总分(即基本要求得分和相应申报等级基本条件得分之和)及实地考察情况上报等级评定委员会。

7.2.3 评定

7.2.3.1 由评定委员会组织等级评定,评定专家不少于 11 人,并应涵盖医疗、康复、养老、护理、健康管理、养老企业管理等专业人员。

7.2.3.2 申报等级评定的医养结合服务机构的"医养结合服务机构等级评定内容及分值"基本要求和基本条件实际得分之和应不低于总分的 80%。

7.2.3.3 申报单位现场答辩,评定专家现场无记名投票表决。

7.2.3.4 评定结果的确定,评定结果分为:通过、暂缓通过、不通过 3 种情况。

a) 评定结果为"通过"。经等级评定委员会评定通过的医养结合服务机构,由中国老年医学学会授予相应的医养结合服务机构等级证书及牌匾,有效期为3年(自颁发证书之日起计算)。

b) 评定结果为"暂缓通过"。经等级评定委员会评定为暂缓通过的医养结合服务机构不授予医养结合服务机构等级证书及牌匾,申报单位可在下一年度重新申报。

c) 评定结果为"不通过"。经等级评定委员会评定为不通过的医养结合服务机构不授予医养结合服务机构等级证书及牌匾,申报单位可在下一年度可重新申报。

d) 经过等级认定的医养结合服务机构可在下一年度申请更高等级的评定,其评定程序与首次评定相同。

7.2.3.5 公示。由等级评定委员会在中国老年医学学会官网发布,公示无异议则由等级评定委员会公布评定结果。

7.2.4 复审与申诉

a) 医养结合服务机构获得评定等级后1年内,评定委员会应派出专家复审组对已评定等级的单位进行复审,复审中发现有与申报不符或出现明显服务质量问题并造成社会影响的,应根据情节作如下处理:书面警告、通报批评、降低等级直至取消等级并收回等级标识。

b) 评定等级被取消后3年内不得申请。

c) 申报单位对评定过程、评定结果有异议时可向中国老年医学学会提出申诉,中国老年医学学会在接到申诉书的30天内应给予明确回复。

附　录　A
（规范性附录）
医养结合服务机构等级评定内容与分值

A.1　医养结合服务机构等级评定内容与分值:基本要求(见表 A.1)。

表 A.1　医养结合服务机构等级评定内容与分值:基本要求

评定项目	总分值	评定内容	分项分值	优秀	良好	一般	较差
基本要求							
建筑与环境	100	绿化面积	10	10～8	7～5	4～2	1～0
		建筑布局	10	10～8	7～5	4～2	1～0
		交通便捷度	10	10～8	7～5	4～2	1～0
		公共信息图形表示	10	10～8	7～5	4～2	1～0
		院内无障碍通道	20	20～15	14～9	8～4	3～0
		室内温度	15	15～12	11～7	6～3	2～0
		室内自然光照	15	15～12	11～7	6～3	2～0
		停车空间	10	10～8	7～5	4～2	1～0
设施设备	300	居室空间	20	20～15	14～9	8～4	3～0
		卫生洗浴空间	15	15～12	11～7	6～3	2～0
		餐厅空间	20	20～15	14～9	8～4	3～0
		休闲活动场所	20	20～15	14～9	8～4	3～0
		康复用房	30	30～22	21～13	12～4	3～0
		康复器械	30	30～22	21～13	12～4	3～0
		医务室用房	30	30～22	21～13	12～4	3～0
		医疗设备(6.2.1.2要求)	30	30～22	21～13	12～4	3～0
		护理站空间	30	30～22	21～13	12～4	3～0
		地面防滑、防跌倒设施	20	20～15	14～9	8～4	3～0
		器械防伤害处理	20	20～15	14～9	8～4	3～0
		洗涤、消毒间	15	15～12	11～7	6～3	2～0
		污物处理	20	20～15	14～9	8～4	3～0
运营管理	100	医疗、养老机构执业证明	10	10～8	7～5	4～2	1～0
		房产证明	10	10～8	7～5	4～2	1～0
		消防、食品卫生经营许可	10	10～8	7～5	4～2	1～0
		特种设备使用登记、许可	10	10～8	7～5	4～2	1～0
		服务人员资质(6.1.3要求)	20	20～15	14～9	8～4	3～0
		管理制度(6.1.4要求)	30	30～22	21～13	12～4	3～0
		评价与改进	10	10～8	7～5	4～2	1～0

A.2 一级医养结合服务机构等级评定内容与分值:基本条件(见表 A.2)。

表 A.2 一级医养结合服务机构等级评定内容与分值:基本条件

评定项目	总分值	评定内容	分项分值	优秀	良好	一般	较差
基本条件	500	医养结合机构规模	10	10～8	7～5	4～2	1～0
		自建医疗机构	10	10～8	7～5	4～2	1～0
		依托或协议医院	10	10～8	7～5	4～2	1～0
		护理/养老人数比例	10	10～8	7～5	4～2	1～0
		专业职称养老护理人员比例	10	10～8	7～5	4～2	1～0
		机构入住率	20	20～15	14～9	8～4	3～0
		出入院服务	10	10～8	7～5	4～2	1～0
		生活照料服务	100	100～80	79～50	49～20	19～0
		养老老人年度查体服务	10	10～8	7～5	4～2	1～0
		膳食服务	10	10～8	7～5	4～2	1～0
		清洁卫生服务	10	10～8	7～5	4～2	1～0
		洗涤服务	10	10～8	7～5	4～2	1～0
		理发服务	10	10～8	7～5	4～2	1～0
		心理咨询服务	10	10～8	7～5	4～2	1～0
		护理服务	70	70～50	49～30	29～13	12～0
		康复治疗服务	70	70～50	49～30	29～13	12～0
		医疗服务	80	80～60	59～36	35～16	15～0
		医疗与养老衔接满意度	10	10～8	7～5	4～2	1～0
		办公网络	10	10～8	7～5	4～2	1～0
		出院后随访	10	10～8	7～5	4～2	1～0
		服务质量评价与改进	10	10～8	7～5	4～2	1～0

A.3 二级医养结合服务机构等级评定内容与分值:基本条件(见表 A.3)。

表 A.3 二级医养结合服务机构等级评定内容与分值:基本条件

评定项目	总分值	评定内容	分项分值	优秀	良好	一般	较差
基本条件	700	医养结合机构规模	20	20～15	14～9	8～4	3～0
		自建医疗机构	20	20～15	14～9	8～4	3～0
		依托或协议医院	10	10～8	7～5	4～2	1～0
		护理/养老人数比例	20	20～15	14～9	8～4	3～0
		专业职称养老护理人员比例	20	20～15	14～9	8～4	3～0
		机构入住率	20	20～15	14～9	8～4	3～0

表 A.3（续）

评定项目	总分值	评定内容	分项分值	优秀	良好	一般	较差
基本条件	700	出入院服务	10	10～8	7～5	4～2	1～0
		生活照料服务	100	100～80	79～50	49～20	19～0
		养老老人年度查体服务	10	10～8	7～5	4～2	1～0
		膳食服务	10	10～8	7～5	4～2	1～0
		清洁卫生服务	10	10～8	7～5	4～2	1～0
		洗涤服务	10	10～8	7～5	4～2	1～0
		理发服务	10	10～8	7～5	4～2	1～0
		代购代邮服务	10	10～8	7～5	4～2	1～0
		通信服务	10	10～8	7～5	4～2	1～0
		文化娱乐服务	10	10～8	7～5	4～2	1～0
		心理/精神支持服务	20	20～15	14～9	8～4	3～0
		安宁疗护服务	30	30～22	21～13	12～4	3～0
		营养评估服务	10	10～8	7～5	4～2	1～0
		护理服务	80	80～60	59～36	35～16	15～0
		康复治疗服务	80	80～60	59～36	35～16	15～0
		医疗服务	100	100～80	79～50	49～20	19～0
		医疗与养老衔接满意度	30	30～22	21～13	12～4	3～0
		办公网络	10	10～8	7～5	4～2	1～0
		视频网络化院外会诊服务	20	20～15	14～9	8～4	3～0
		出院后随访	10	10～8	7～5	4～2	1～0
		服务质量评价与改进	10	10～8	7～5	4～2	1～0

A.4 三级医养结合服务机构等级评定内容与分值:基本条件(见表 A.4)。

表 A.4 三级医养结合服务机构等级评定内容与分值:基本条件

评定项目	总分值	评定内容	分项分值	优秀	良好	一般	较差
基本条件	900	医养结合机构规模	30	30～22	21～13	12～4	3～0
		自建医疗机构	30	30～22	21～13	12～4	3～0
		依托或协议医院	20	20～15	14～9	8～4	3～0
		护理/养老人数比例	30	30～22	21～13	12～4	3～0
		专业职称养老护理人员比例	30	30～22	21～13	12～4	3～0
		机构入住率	30	30～22	21～13	12～4	3～0
		出入院服务	10	10～8	7～5	4～2	1～0

表 A.4（续）

评定项目	总分值	评定内容	分项分值	优秀	良好	一般	较差
基本条件	900	生活照料服务	100	100～80	79～50	49～20	19～0
		养老老年人年度查体服务	10	10～8	7～5	4～2	1～0
		膳食服务	10	10～8	7～5	4～2	1～0
		清洁卫生服务	10	10～8	7～5	4～2	1～0
		洗涤服务	10	10～8	7～5	4～2	1～0
		理发服务	10	10～8	7～5	4～2	1～0
		代购代邮服务	10	10～8	7～5	4～2	1～0
		通信服务	10	10～8	7～5	4～2	1～0
		文化娱乐服务	10	10～8	7～5	4～2	1～0
		体育健身服务	10	10～8	7～5	4～2	1～0
		旅游服务	10	10～8	7～5	4～2	1～0
		心理/精神支持服务	20	20～15	14～9	8～4	3～0
		安宁疗护服务	30	30～22	21～13	12～4	3～0
		舒缓医疗服务	30	30～22	21～13	12～4	3～0
		营养评估服务	10	10～8	7～5	4～2	1～0
		护理服务	80	80～60	59～36	35～16	15～0
		康复治疗服务	80	80～60	59～36	35～16	15～0
		中医康复、养生	80	80～60	59～36	35～16	15～0
		医疗服务	100	100～80	79～50	49～20	19～0
		医疗与养老衔接满意度	30	30～22	21～13	12～4	3～0
		办公网络	10	10～8	7～5	4～2	1～0
		视频网络化院外会诊服务	20	20～15	14～9	8～4	3～0
		出院后随访	10	10～8	7～5	4～2	1～0
		社会工作者服务	10	10～8	7～5	4～2	1～0
		服务质量评价与改进	10	10～8	7～5	4～2	1～0

A.5 四级医养结合服务机构等级评定内容与分值：基本条件（见表 A.5）。

表 A.5 四级医养结合服务机构等级评定内容与分值：基本条件

评定项目	总分值	评定内容	分项分值	优秀	良好	一般	较差
基本条件	1 000	医养结合机构规模	40	40～30	29～18	17～8	7～0
		自建医疗机构	40	40～30	29～18	17～8	7～0
		依托或协议医院	20	20～15	14～9	8～4	3～0

表 A.5（续）

评定项目	总分值	评定内容	分项分值	优秀	良好	一般	较差
基本条件	1 000	护理/养老人数比例	40	40～30	29～18	17～8	7～0
		专业职称养老护理人员比例	40	40～30	29～18	17～8	7～0
		机构入住率	40	40～30	29～18	17～8	7～0
		出入院服务	10	10～8	7～5	4～2	1～0
		生活照料服务	100	100～80	79～50	49～20	19～0
		养老老人年度查体服务	10	10～8	7～5	4～2	1～0
		膳食服务	10	10～8	7～5	4～2	1～0
		清洁卫生服务	10	10～8	7～5	4～2	1～0
		洗涤服务	10	10～8	7～5	4～2	1～0
		理发服务	10	10～8	7～5	4～2	1～0
		代购代邮服务	10	10～8	7～5	4～2	1～0
		通信服务	10	10～8	7～5	4～2	1～0
		文化、娱乐服务	10	10～8	7～5	4～2	1～0
		老年大学	10	10～8	7～5	4～2	1～0
		体育健身服务	10	10～8	7～5	4～2	1～0
		旅游服务	10	10～8	7～5	4～2	1～0
		心理/精神支持服务	20	20～15	14～9	8～4	3～0
		安宁疗护服务	30	30～22	21～13	12～4	3～0
		舒缓医疗服务	30	30～22	21～13	12～4	3～0
		营养评估服务	10	10～8	7～5	4～2	1～0
		护理服务	80	80～60	59～36	35～16	15～0
		康复治疗服务	80	80～60	59～36	35～16	15～0
		中医康复、养生	80	80～60	59～36	35～16	15～0
		医疗服务	100	100～80	79～50	49～20	19～0
		家庭签约服务	30	30～22	21～13	12～4	3～0
		医疗与养老衔接满意度	30	30～22	21～13	12～4	3～0
		办公网络化服务	10	10～8	7～5	4～2	1～0
		地区权威医院网络化会诊	30	30～22	21～13	12～4	3～0
		出院后随访	10	20～15	14～9	8～4	3～0
		社会工作者服务	10	10～8	7～5	4～2	1～0
		服务质量评价与改进	10	10～8	7～5	4～2	1～0

A.6 五级医养结合服务机构等级评定内容与分值:基本条件(见表 A.6)。

表 A.6 五级医养结合服务机构等级评定内容与分值:基本条件

评定项目	总分值	评定内容	分项分值	优秀	良好	一般	较差
基本条件	1 100	医养结合机构规模	50	50～40	39～25	24～10	9～0
		自建医疗机构	50	50～40	39～25	24～10	9～0
		依托或协议医院	30	30～22	21～13	12～4	3～0
		护理/养老人人数比例	50	50～40	39～25	24～10	9～0
		专业职称养护人数比例	50	50～40	39～25	24～10	9～0
		机构入住率	50	50～40	39～25	24～10	9～0
		出入院服务	10	10～8	7～5	4～2	1～0
		生活照料服务	100	100～80	79～50	49～20	19～0
		养老老人年度查体服务	20	20～15	14～9	8～4	3～0
		膳食服务	10	10～8	7～5	4～2	1～0
		清洁卫生服务	10	10～8	7～5	4～2	1～0
		洗涤服务	10	10～8	7～5	4～2	1～0
		理发服务	10	10～8	7～5	4～2	1～0
		购物、代购服务	10	10～8	7～5	4～2	1～0
		通信、邮电、代邮服务	10	10～8	7～5	4～2	1～0
		文化、娱乐服务	10	10～8	7～5	4～2	1～0
		老年大学	10	10～8	7～5	4～2	1～0
		体育健身服务	10	10～8	7～5	4～2	1～0
		旅游、社交服务	10	10～8	7～5	4～2	1～0
		种植园艺服务	10	10～8	7～5	4～2	1～0
		心理/精神支持服务	30	30～22	21～13	12～4	3～0
		安宁疗护服务	30	30～22	21～13	12～4	3～0
		舒缓医疗服务	30	30～22	21～13	12～4	3～0
		营养评估、指导膳食服务	20	20～15	14～9	8～4	3～0
		护理服务	80	80～60	59～36	35～16	15～0
		康复治疗服务	80	80～60	59～36	35～16	15～0
		中医康复、养生	70	70～50	49～30	29～13	12～0
		医疗服务	100	100～80	79～50	49～20	19～0
		家庭签约服务	30	30～22	21～13	12～4	3～0
		医疗与养老衔接满意度	30	30～22	21～13	12～4	3～0
		办公网络化服务	10	10～8	7～5	4～2	1～0
		国内权威医院网络化会诊	30	30～22	21～13	12～4	3～0

表 A.6（续）

评定项目	总分值	评定内容	分项分值	优秀	良好	一般	较差
基本条件	1 100	出院后随访	20	20～15	14～9	8～4	3～0
		社会工作者服务	10	10～8	7～5	4～2	1～0
		服务质量评价与改进	20	20～15	14～9	8～4	3～0

参 考 文 献

［1］ 《综合医院分级护理指导原则(试行)》A3ZDYY-NY-20070924055 国家卫生部

［2］ 《护理院基本标准(2011 版)》国家卫生部

［3］ 《医疗机构从业人员行为规范》(2012)国家卫生部

［4］ 《养老机构医务室基本标准(试行)》(2014)国家卫计委

［5］ 《养老机构护理站基本标准(试行)》(2014)国家卫计委

［6］ 《国家基本公共卫生服务规范(第 3 版)》(2017)国家卫计委

［7］ 《老年友善医院规范》T/CGSS 003—2018 中国老年医学学会

ICS 03.080.99
A 20

Social Organization Standard

T/CGSS 006—2019

Grade assessment specification for service institutions of combination of medical and senior health care

医养结合服务机构等级评定规范

（English Translation）

Issue date：2019-04-28

Implementation date：2019-04-28

Issued by Chinese Geriatrics Society

Foreword

This standard was drafted in accordance with the rules given in GB/T 1. 1—2009.

This standard was proposed by Department of Integrated Medical and Nursing Management and Department of Standardization Management of Chinese Geriatric Society.

This standed was prepared by Chinese Geriatrics Society.

This standard was drafted by Promotion Committee of Medical Care Integration of Chinese Geriatrics Society,Chinese PLA General Hospital,National Clinical Research Center of Geriatrics Disease(Chinese PLA General Hospital),Institute of Architectural Environmental Art Design of China IPPR International Engineering Co. , Ltd. ,Liaoning Zhongzhi Shengjing Hospital of Geriatrics, Qingcheng International Care Center of Chengdu in Sichuan Province, Xinhexin Health and Senior Care Investment Limited Company of Guilin in Guangxi, Kaixuan Elderly Hospital of Linyi in Shandong Province,; Health Committee of Shenyang, the Fifth Affiliated Hospital of Zhengzhou University, the Eighth People's Hospital of Chengdu in Sichuan Province, the Third People's Hospital of Gansu Province, the Second People's Hospital of Changzhi in Shanxi Province, Binzhou Medical College of Shandong Province, and Home for the Aged Guangzhou.

The main drafters of this standard were Tingshu Yang,Zongyao Long, Shengqiang Jiao, Qun Wang, Feng Lin, Zhijun Sun, Qiang Wu, Lihong Cheng, Changchun Yang,Huiru Hou,YaogaiLi,Weihua Xu, Yafei Zhang, Kaitian Jiang, Pengyuan Zheng, Hailang Huang,Liping Lu, Buqing Wang, Yuling Hao, Lianqi Liu, Liannong Xiao, Shao Chen and Dongke Li.

Introduction

The current population above the age of 60 in China is about 250 million. Population has been aging and the number of empty nesters has been increasing. Thus, the number of elder populations with disabilities has been continuously increasing, potentially resulting in the imbalance between the high demand and limited supply of care services.

The 19th national congress of the Communist Party of China addresses that the health level of a population is an important indicator of the prosperity level of a society and a nation. The government will take proactive measures for population aging issues, create a supportive and respectful environment and adopt policies designed for offering elderly care services, elderly-friendly services, and engaging medical services with elderly care services and focus on developing healthcare industry for aging population. The Government Work Report published at the Second Session of the Thirteenth National People's Congress of the People's Republic of China, also addresses the focus on developing elderly care services, especially community-based elderly care services, and indicates that we will strive to reform and improve the health policies for engaging medical services with the elderly care services, so that the elderly will enjoy a happy life in their later years.

At present, a variety of care service institutions have developed rapidly and been providing services in China. A new form of care provider that combines medical service and elderly care services has been growing widely across the nation, with various functions such as medical care, elderly care and rehabilitation care. To further develop, manage and regulate such care providing institutions, this standard provides grade assessment specification for service institutions of combination of medical and senior health care.

Grade assessment specification for service institutions of combination of medical and senior health care

1 Scope

This standard specifies the assessment criteria and grade standards, basic requirements and conditions for grading application as well as organization and management for grading assessment for service institutions of combination of medical and senior health care.

This standard is applicable to the assessment and grade evaluation of service institutions of combination of medical and senior health care.

2 Normative references

The following referenced documents are indispensable for the application of this document. For dated references, only the edition cited applies. For undated references, the latest edition of the referenced document (including any amendments) applies.

GB/T 29353   Basic standards for senior care organization

GB/T 37276   Classification and accreditation for senior care organization

GB 35796   Basic specifications of service quality for senior care organization

MZ/T 039   Capability assessment of the elderly

JGJ 450   Standards for architectural design of elderly care service facilities

T/CGSS 001   Specification for elderly caregiver

T/CGSS 005   Basic requirements of infrastructure for service institutions of combination of medical and senior health care

3 Terms and definitions

For the purposes of this document, the terms and definitions given in GB/T 37276, T/CGSS 005 and the following apply.

3. 1

service institutions of combination of medical and senior health care

an institution with both medical and elderly care qualifications and capabilities to combinedly provide medical and elderly care services as well as health management services
［T/CGSS 005—2009,definition 3. 1］

3. 2

grade

a classification based on a comprehensive assessment of the environment, facilities, equipments, operation, management and service qualityof elderly care institutions

3. 3

occupancy rate

the ratio of the total number of elderly residents to the total number of beds in a care service institution（％）

3. 4

medical care services

activities to provide basic medical treatment, prevention, health care, rehabilitation and health management in elderly care institutions

3. 5

nursing services

licensed practicing nurses provide diagnosis and treatment for existing or potential health problems of the elderly according to general rules of nursing care, and provide instructions for nurse practitioners and caregivers to complete independently tasks of daily care service, basic nursing practice and psychological counseling service for the elderly

4 General principles

4. 1   Grade assessment shall be comprehensive and objective, quality oriented, pragmatic, just and fair to ensure the credibility of the assessment results.

4. 2   The basic requirements and basic conditions are the key elements in grading evaluation. The basic requirements are the criteria for grading assessment,and the basic conditions are the standards used to determine the grade level.

4. 3 An important indicator of grade evaluation is the infrastructure and service contents shall be a-dapted to service area, service population, and service needs. The focus should be on elderly care, health protection, rehabilitation and health preservation, and service content and service quality should be emphasized.

5 Classification of grade

5. 1 Scale classification of service institutions of combination of medical and senior health care

5. 1. 1 The sacle classification of hospitalsshall be implemented according to the *Classification andmanagement standards of comphrehensive hospitals* (*A3ZDYY-NY*-20070924055) issued by the former of National Ministry of Health

5. 1. 2 The medical and nursing institutions can be classified into three groups: large-sized, medi-um-sized and small-sized (see Table 1)

Table 1 Size of medical and nursing service institutions

institution	the number of beds		
	large-sized	medium-sized	small-sized
nursing home	≥501	151～500	≤150
nursing home for the elderly	≥301	101～300	≤100
day care center for the aged	≥101	51～100	≤50

5. 2 Grade of service institutions of combination of medical and senior health care

5. 2. 1 Grade levels

There are 5 grade levels of service institutions of combination of medical and senior health care based on their scale and capabilities. Five grade levels ranking from the lowest to the highest are: grade-1, grade-2, grade-3, grade-4 and grade-5. The higher grade indicates larger size of the institu-te, better equipment and more facilities, higher quality of environment and layout design as well as the higher quality of operation, management and services.

5. 2. 2 Grade identification

The grade logo is composed of a number of (up to 5) five-pointed stars. The number of five-pointed stars represent the grade level (from grade 1 to grade 5).

Example: The logo of a five-star (grade 5) service institutions of combination of medical and senior health care,see Figure 1.

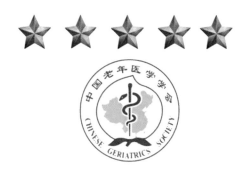

中 国 老 年 医 学 学 会 制

Figure 1 Grade identification

6 Basic requirements and conditions for grading application

6.1 Basic requirements for grading application

6.1.1 The facilities and equipments of service institutions of combination of medical and senior health care shall meet the requirements of GB/T 29353 and T/CGSS 005.

6.1.2 Service institutions of combination of medical and senior health care shall have the valid practice licenses as below：

a) Any elderly care institution shall hold "*Approval Certificate for the Establishment of Social Welfare Institutions*", valid "*Business license*" or "*Certificate of the Legal Person of Public Institutions*" or "*Registration Certificate of Civilian-run non-Enterprise Units*", and medical institutions shall have a "*Medical Institution Practice License*".

b) Property lien or lease agreement，fire inspection certificate or fire protection document.

c) Institutions providing catering service shall have a food hygiene license.

d) Institutions using special equipments shall have the corresponding registration certificates for the use of special equipments，including，but not limited to，the registration certificate for the use of elevators and boilers，etc.

6.1.3 Qualifications of personnel in service institutions of combination of medical and senior health care：

a) Physicians in medical and nursing service institutions shall hold "*Medical Doctor Qualification Certificate*" and "*Medical Practice Certificate*", nurses shall hold "*Nurse Practice Certificate*", other professionals shall hold appropriate professional qualification certificates and practice certificates. Geriatric caregivers and/or senior caregivers shall meet the relevant national regulations and T/CGSS 001 requirements or be qualified upon the completion of professional training.

b） All staff members shall have health certificates.

6.1.4 The management system shall be in accordance with the requirements given in GB/T 35796, including but not limited to:

a） Office management system,

b） In and out patient management and follow-up system,

c） Service management and quality control system,

d） Medical consultation system,

e） Surveillance system of medical operations,

f） Health management and medical record system,

g） Emergency on-duty system,

h） Two-way referrals and "green channel" (express channel) in medical and nursing institutions,

i） Information management system,

j） Human resource management system,

k） Financial management and special fund management system,

l） Logistics management system,

m） Safety management system, including, but not limited to, food safety management system, facilities and equipment safety management system,

n） Medical waste management system.

6.1.5 The basic requirements of assessment and grading contents of service institutions of combination of medical and senior health careare specified in Table A.1.

6.2 The basic conditions for grading application

6.2.1 Grade-1 service institutions of combination of medical and senior health care

6.2.1.1 Medical and care institutions shall meet the construction standards of "small-sized" institution according to 5.1.1.

6.2.1.2 Care institutions shall have infirmaries and nursing stations which shall meet the requirements of *Basic Standards of infirmary of in ederly care institutions* (trial)(2014) and *Basic standards of nursing stations* in elderly *care institutions* (trial)(2014) by the former National Health and Family Planning Commission.

6.2.1.3 Operation management shall meet all requirements in 6.1.

6.2.1.4 The allocation of nursing staff in senior care institutions shall meet the requirements of GB/T 35796 and GB/T 37276. Each nursing unit shall be staffed with at least 1 nurse and 1 nurse supervisor with professional certificates of senior caregiver.

6.2.1.5 No less than 50% of the personnel in senior care institutions hold entry-level (and above) elderly caregiver certificates and /or have been trained to meet requirements for entry-level caregivers.

6.2.1.6 The occupancy rate of care institutions shall meet the requirements of GB/T 37276. The occupancy rate of care institution for the elderly with disabilities shall not be less than 30%.

6.2.1.7 Service contents of senior care institutions shall include items according to GB/T 29353. In addition, service contents shall also include in and out patient service, capability assessment for the elderly, daily service, medical care service, annual physical examination service, psychological counseling service, dietary service, cleaning service, laundry service and haircut service, etc.

6.2.1.8 The service quality of senior care institutions shall meet the requirements of GB 35796.

6.2.1.9 Senior care institutions shall have information technology system including but not limited to inter-office network system, health management network for the elderly, hospital discharge and follow-up network system.

6.2.1.10 No liability accident shall have ever happened within the recent 1a. The service quality satisfaction rate shall be above 85%, and a service improvement plan shall be in place.

6.2.1.11 The assessment contents and grading levels of grade-1 service institutions of combination of medical and senior health care are shown in Table A.2.

6.2.2 Grade-2 service institutions of combination of medical and senior health care

6.2.2.1 Grade-2 service institutions of combination of medical and senior health care shall at least meet the requirements of 6.2.1.

6.2.2.2 Satisfying the "small-sized" construction standards defined in 5.1.1, the construction design of grade-2 service institutions of combination of medical and senior health care shall include supermarket, post-office, haircut and other facilities providing comprehensive services.

6.2.2.3 The ratio of nursing staff to the elderly in senior care institutions shall be according to grade-2 care institutions in GB/T 37276.

6.2.2.4 The proportion of personnel who hold the certificates of caregiver of entry-level or above or who have been trained to meet the standard of entry-level caregiver shall not be less than 60%.

6.2.2.5 The occupancy rate of senior care institutions shall be according to grade-2 care institutions in GB/T 37276. The occupancy rate of care institutions for the elderly with disabilities shall not be less than 30%.

6.2.2.6 Service contents shall be according to 6.2.1.7. Additional services including hospice care service, psychological counseling/emotional support service, nutrition evaluation service, cultural and entertainment service, communication and transportation service, and mailing service, etc. shall be provided.

6.2.2.7 Information technology system shall be according to 6.2.1.9. In addition, grade-2 care service institution shall be capable of providingvideonetwork consultation systemwith experts from service institutions of combination of medical and senior health care.

6.2.2.8 No liability accident shall have ever happened within the recent 1a. The service quality satisfaction rate shall be above 90%,and a service improvement plan shall be in place.

6.2.2.9 The assessment contents and grading levels of grade-2 service institutions of combination of medical and senior health care are specified in Table A.3.

6.2.3 Grade-3 service institutions of combination of medical and senior health care

6.2.3.1 Grade-3 service institutions of combination of medical and senior health care shall at least meet the requirements of 6.2.2.

6.2.3.2 Satisfying the "medium-sized" construction standards defined in 5.1.1, the construction design of grade-2 service institutions of combination of medical and senior health care shall also have sports activity room, entertainment room, beauty room and other comprehensive service facilities. The residential housing shall be equipped with refrigerators, colored televisions, etc.

6.2.3.3 Grade-3 service institutions of combination of medical and senior health care shall have self-built graded comprehensive hospital or rehabilitation institutions (level II or above) or have established agreements with adjacent level II or above comprehensive (rehabilitation) hospitals to share medical resource, and have established "green channels" (express channel) for medical referrals and critical medical conditions.

6.2.3.4 Each nursing unit within senior care institutions shall have medical clinics and nursing stations.

6.2.3.5 Old people's home and nursing homes for the elderly shall have hospice nursing rooms constructed relatively in isolation yet adjacent to infirmary. The entrance of hospice nursing shall not be merged with the entrance of residential facilities for the elderly.

6.2.3.6 The ratio of the number of nursing staff to the number of the elderly residents in senior care institutions shall be according to grade-3 care institutions in GB/T 37276.

6.2.3.7 The allocation of medical staff in nursing homes for the elderly shall follow the *Basic Standards of Nursing homes* （2011） issued by the former Ministry of Health.

6.2.3.8 The proportion of personnel who hold the certificates of caregiver of entry-level or above or who have been trained to meet the standard of entry-level caregivers shall not be less than 70%.

6.2.3.9 The occupancy rate of senior care institutions shall meet the requirements of GB/T 37276 defined for grade-3 senior care institutions. The occupancy rate of care institutions for the elderly with disabilities shall not be less than 30%.

6.2.3.10 Service contents shall be according to 6.2.2.6. Additional services including soothing care，Chinese medicine health care，health care services，sports，culture，entertainment，tourism services etc. shall be provided.

6.2.3.11 Information technology system shall be according to 6.2.2.7. In addition，network connection with other major hospitals and medical institutions shall be established. "Green channel" （express channel） shall be provided for clinical and treatment consultations for patients with severe illnesses and conditions.

6.2.3.12 At least 1 social worker in charge of social work management in senior care institutions is required.

6.2.3.13 No liability accident shall have ever happened within the recent 1a. The service quality satisfaction rate shall be above 95%，and a service improvement plan shall be in place.

6.2.3.14 The assessment contents and grading levels for grade-3 service institutions of combination of medical and senior health care are specified in Table A.4.

6.2.4 Grade-4 service institutions of combination of medical and senior health care

6.2.4.1 Grade-4 service institutions of combination of medical and senior health care shall at least meet the requirements in 6. 2. 3.

6. 2. 4. 2   Satisfying the "large-sized" construction standards defined in 5. 1. 1, the organization shall have fully completed infrastructure, high degree of modernization, capability of providing comprehensive services, excellent service quality, comfortable indoor environment and beautiful outdoor environment.

6. 2. 4. 3   The infrastructure of medical facilities shall meet the requirements of 6. 2. 3. 3. The institutions shall have established collaborative relationships with local or domestic hospitals with high reputation, and strive to improve continuously the quality and capability of care through technical communication and talent development plans.

6. 2. 4. 4   The ratio of the number of nursing staff to the number of the elderly residents in senior care institutions shall be according to grade-4 care institutions in GB/T 37276.

6. 2. 4. 5   The proportion of personnel who hold the certificates of caregiver of entry-level or above or who have been trained to meet the standard of entry-level caregivers shall not be less than 80%.

6. 2. 4. 6   The occupancy rate of senior care institutions shall meet the requirements in GB/T 37276 defined for grade-4 senior care institutions. The occupancy rate of care institutions for the elderly with disabilities shall not be less than 30%.

6. 2. 4. 7   Each nursing unit within senior care institutions shall have independent medical clinics and nursing stations.

6. 2. 4. 8   In addition to be according to 6. 2. 3. 10, grade-4 service institutions shall provide elderly university program and contracted domestic service providers,etc.

6. 2. 4. 9   Information technology system shall be according to 6. 2. 3. 11. In addition, network connection with other major hospitals and medical institution shall be established for video conferencing to provide medical consultation, consultation services for patients with severe and difficult conditions as well as assistance and guidance for emergency rescues and major surgeries.

6. 2. 4. 10   At least 1~2 social workers in charge of social work management in senior care institutions shall be available.

6. 2. 4. 11   No liability accident shall have ever happened within the recent 1a. The service quality satisfaction rate shall be above 95% and a service improvement plan shall bein place.

6. 2. 4. 12   Assessment contents and grading levels for grade-4 service institutions of combination of medical and senior health care are specified in Table A. 5.

6.2.5 Grade-5 service institutions of combination of medical and senior health care

6.2.5.1 Grade-5 service institutions of combination of medical and senior health care shall at least meet the requirements in 6.2.4.

6.2.5.2 Satisfying the "large-sized" construction standards defined in 5.1.1, the organization shall have great ecological environment, fully-equipped facilities, up to date equipment, full and high-quality services. It shall also provide social, tourism, entertainment, shopping, leisure, culture, art, health and fitness and other activities.

6.2.5.3 The ratio of the number of nursing staff to the number of the elderly residents in senior care institutions should shall be according to grade-5 care institutions in GB/T 37276.

6.2.5.4 The occupancy rate of senior care institutions shall be according to grade-5 care institutions in GB/T 37276. The occupancy rate of care institution for the elderly with disabilities shall not be less than 30%.

6.2.5.5 In addition to services specified in 6.2.4.8, grade-5 service institutions shall provide gardening services, art education services, social activities, financial services and legal services, etc.

6.2.5.6 Information technology system shall be according to 6.2.4.9. In addition, video network connection with other well-known medical institutions shall be established to provide medical consultation services.

6.2.5.7 At least two social workers in charge of social work management in senior care institutions shall be available.

6.2.5.8 Assessment contents and grading levels for grade-5 service institutions of combination of medical and senior health care are specified in Table A.6.

7 Grading organization andmanagement

7.1 Composition and duties of the assessment committee

Chinese Geriatric Society has established the assessment committee of service institutions of combination of medical and senior health care("assessment committee") ,managing and coordinating nationwide assessment and grading of service institutions of combination of medical and senior health care.

7.2 Grading process and methods

7.2.1 Process flow

The flow chart of grading assessment of service institutions of combination of medical and senior health care is shown in Figure 2.

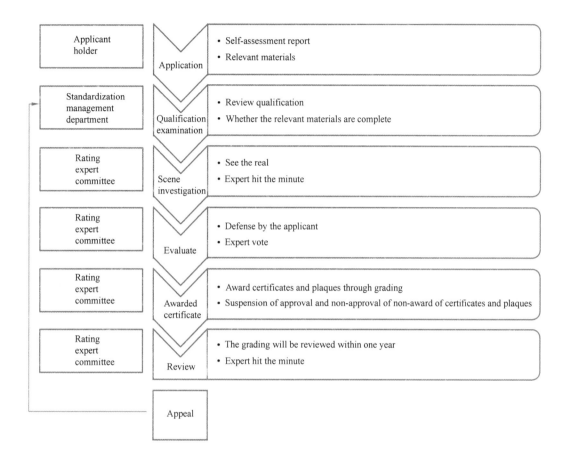

Figure 2　Flow chart of review and grading medical and nursing service institutions

7.2.2　Method

7.2.2.1　Application

Service institutions of combination of medical and senior health care should apply voluntarily for grading assessment at Department of Standardization Management of Chinese Geriatric Society through the submission of self-evaluation reports and other relevant materials. The application materials shall include:

a)　*Approval for the Establishment of Social Welfare institutions* and *Business License of Social Welfare institutions* of service institutions of combination of medical and senior health care (such as senior nursing homes, care centers, and day care center for the aged).

b)　*Medical Institution Practice License of* self-built medical unit (such as general hospital, rehabilitation hospital or specialist hospital, infirmary/out-patient department).

c)　Collaboration agreement between the care service organization and the dependent medical service entities as well as *Medicall nstitution Practice License* of the cooperative medical service entities (such as medical service unit or hospitals).

d) Self-evaluation report of the applicant shall include the following items:

    1) The scale of the medical and nursing service organization shall be definedclearly, and the grade level of the application to be assessed for shall be definedclearly.

    2) Equipment and devices available for elderly care service, rehabilitation service and medical service provided at the institution.

    3) The infrastructure and management plan for medical service, medical technology, nursing service, care service, logistics and talent management of the institution.

    4) The evaluation of a pilot operation of the institution focusing on social and economic benefits, quality assessment, satisfaction rate and improvement plans.

e) Upon any following conducts, the institution will be disqualified for any in-progress grading assessment:

    1) Any major violations of law, discipline and regulations.

    2) Any violations of grading assessment disciplines. Any behaviors impairing the fairness and equality of the grading assessment. Any interference with the grading assessment.

    3) Submitting false material on purpose, faking assessment materials, providing fraudulent information.

    4) Any major misconduct of medical ethics, medical quality and medical safety.

7.2.2.2 Qualification examination

Department of Standardization Management of Chinese Geriatric Society shall, within 20 business days upon receipt of the application materials, conduct a qualification examination on the application materials of the applicant units, including:

a) The operation certificates the medical and elderly care service institutions shall comply with the relevant state provisions. Document of certificates (photocopies) shall be submitted.

b) The applicant unit shall meet the qualifications defined in 7.2.2.1.

c) Three outcomes will be determined based on the qualification examination: approval, revisit after supplement materials submission or disapproval.

7.2.2.3 Field investigation

a) The assessment committee consist of more than 5 experts (field investigation committee) shall conduct a field visit at the applicant institute.

b) The field investigation committee shall make the evaluation based on the final scores according to "assessment and grading criteria for service institutions of combination of medical and enior health care" (see Annex A).

c) The field investigation committee shall report the final score based on "assessment and grading criteria for service institutions of combination of medical and enior health care" to the assessment committee as well as any observations made from the field visit.

7.2.3 Evaluation

7.2.3.1 The assessment committee shall conduct the evaluation process. There shall be no less than 11 subject matter experts from relevant fields such as medical treatment, rehabilitation, senior care, nursing, health management, elderly care service industry and other relevant professions.

7.2.3.2 The actual score evaluated based on both basic requirements and basic conditions of the "assessment and grading criteria for service institutions of combination of medical and enior health care" shall not be less than 80% of the total sum.

7.2.3.3 The applicant unit shall present application in person. The assessment result is determined by anonymous vote of the assessment committee.

7.2.3.4 There are three outcomes of the assessment: approval, suspending approval and disapproval:

a) Approval: The service institutions of combination of medical and enior health care assessed and approved by the assessment committee shall be awarded the corresponding grade certificate by Chinese Geriatric Society. The approved grade level shall be valid for 3 years (starting from the date of issuance of the certificate).

b) Suspending approval: The service institution of combination of medical and enior health care which has been assessed by the assessment but is not granted any grade certificate and will be reassessed the next year.

c) Disapproval: The service institution of combination of medical and enior health care shall not be granted any grade certificate. The applicant unit may re-apply for grade assessment the next year.

d) A service institution of combination of medical and enior health care that has been approved for the assessed grade level may apply for a higher-grade assessment the next year. The assessment procedure is the same as of the previous assessment.

7.2.3.5 Announcement. The grade assessment committee will publish the evaluation results on the official website of Chinese Geriatric Society, and the grade assessment committee will announce the evaluation results without objections.

7.2.4 Review and appeal

a) After one year from the grade approval, the assessment committee shall conduct a field visit by an expert review team. If any inconsistent observation is made from application materials or service quality impairment with a social impact has occurred, the following treatment shall be applied: official warning, notification of misconduct, downgrade or withdrawn of any grade level.

b) No application shall be made within 3 a after the grade has been withdrawn.

c) If the applicant has any objection to the assessment process and results, it may file a complaint with Chinese Geriatric Society, and Chinese Geriatric Society shall provide the response within 30 d upon receiving the complaint.

Annex A

（Normative）

Assessment and grading criteria for service institutions of combination of medical and enior health care

A. 1   Basic requirements of assessment and grading criteria for service institutions of combination of medical and enior health care are showned in Table A. 1.

Table A. 1   Basic requirements of assessment and grading criteria for
service institutions of combination of medical and enior health care

Evaluation item		Total score	Evaluation content	Score of sub-item	Excellent	Good	General	Poor
Basic requirements	Architecture and environment	100	Landscaping area	10	10～8	7～5	4～2	1～0
			Architectural layout	10	10～8	7～5	4～2	1～0
			Traffic convenience	10	10～8	7～5	4～2	1～0
			Graphical representation of public information	10	10～8	7～5	4～2	1～0
			Barrier-free access in hospital	20	20～15	14～9	8～4	3～0
			Indoor temperature	15	15～12	11～7	6～3	2～0
			Indoor natural light	15	15～12	11～7	6～3	2～0
			Parking space	10	10～8	7～5	4～2	1～0
	facilities and equipment	300	Bedroom space	20	20～15	14～9	8～4	3～0
			Sanitary bath space	15	15～12	11～7	6～3	2～0
			Restaurant space	20	20～15	14～9	8～4	3～0
			Recreational activity place	20	20～15	14～9	8～4	3～0
			Rehabilitation room	30	30～22	21～13	12～4	3～0
			Rehabilitation equipment	30	30～22	21～13	12～4	3～0
			Infirmary room	30	30～22	21～13	12～4	3～0
			Medical equipment（the requirements of 6.2.1.2）	30	30～22	21～13	12～4	3～0
			Nursing station space	30	30～22	21～13	12～4	3～0
			Anti-slippery and fall prevention facilities	20	20～15	14～9	8～4	3～0
			Injury prevention and treatment of equipment	20	20～15	14～9	8～4	3～0
			Laundry and disinfection room	15	15～12	11～7	6～3	2～0
			Sewage treatment	20	20～15	14～9	8～4	3～0

Table A. 1 （*continued*）

Evaluation item		Total score	Evaluation content	Score of sub-item	Excellent	Good	General	Poor
Basic requirements	Operation management	100	License and certificate of medical and senior care institutions	10	10~8	7~5	4~2	1~0
			Real estate certificate	10	10~8	7~5	4~2	1~0
			Permits for fire protection and food safety	10	10~8	7~5	4~2	1~0
			Registration and license for the use of special equipment	10	10~8	7~5	4~2	1~0
			Qualifications of service personnel （the requirements of 6.1.3）	20	20~15	14~9	8~4	3~0
			Management system （the requirements of 6.1.4）	30	30~22	21~13	12~4	3~0
			Evaluation and improvement	10	10~8	7~5	4~2	1~0

A. 2　Basic conditions of assessment and grading criteria for grade-1 service institutions of combination of medical and enior health care are showned in Table A. 2.

Table A. 2　Basic conditions of assessment and grading criteria for grade-1
service institutions of combination of medical and enior health care

Evaluation item	Total score	Evaluation content	Score of sub-item	Excellent	Good	General	Poor
Basic conditions	500	Scale of medical and nursing institutions	10	10~8	7~5	4~2	1~0
		Self-managed medical institution	10	10~8	7~5	4~2	1~0
		Affiliated hospital	10	10~8	7~5	4~2	1~0
		Nurse/patient ratio	10	10~8	7~5	4~2	1~0
		Proportion of nursing staff with professional titles in senior care	10	10~8	7~5	4~2	1~0
		Institutional occupancy rate	20	20~15	14~9	8~4	3~0
		In and out patient service	10	10~8	7~5	4~2	1~0
		Life assistance service	100	100~80	79~50	49~20	19~0
		Annual physical examination service for the elderly	10	10~8	7~5	4~2	1~0
		Dietary service	10	10~8	7~5	4~2	1~0
		Sanitation service	10	10~8	7~5	4~2	1~0
		Laundry service	10	10~8	7~5	4~2	1~0

Table A. 2 （*continued*）

Evaluation item	Total score	Evaluation content	Score of sub-item	Excellent	Good	General	Poor
Basic conditions	500	Haircut service	10	10～8	7～5	4～2	1～0
		Psychological counseling service	10	10～8	7～5	4～2	1～0
		Nursing service	70	70～50	49～30	29～13	12～0
		Rehabilitation service	70	70～50	49～30	29～13	12～0
		Medical service	80	80～60	59～36	35～16	15～0
		Satisfaction on degree of combining medical and senior care services	10	10～8	7～5	4～2	1～0
		Office network	10	10～8	7～5	4～2	1～0
		Follow-up after discharge	10	10～8	7～5	4～2	1～0
		Service quality evaluation and improvement	10	10～8	7～5	4～2	1～0

A. 3　Basic conditions of assessment and grading criteria for grade-2 service institutions of combination of medical and enior health care are showned in Table A. 3.

Table A. 3　Basic conditions of assessment and grading criteria for grade-2 service institutions of combination of medical and enior health care

Evaluation item	Total score	Evaluation content	Score of sub-item	Excellent	Good	General	Poor
Basic conditions	700	Scale of medical and nursing institutions	20	20～15	14～9	8～4	3～0
		Self-managed medical institution	20	20～15	14～9	8～4	3～0
		Affiliated hospital	10	10～8	7～5	4～2	1～0
		Nurse/patient ratio	20	20～15	14～9	8～4	3～0
		Proportion of nursing staff with professional titles in senior care	20	20～15	14～9	8～4	3～0
		Institutional occupancy rate	20	20～15	14～9	8～4	3～0
		In-and-out patient service	10	10～8	7～5	4～2	1～0
		life assistance service	100	100～80	79～50	49～20	19～0
		Annual physical examination service for the elderly	10	10～8	7～5	4～2	1～0
		Dietary service	10	10～8	7～5	4～2	1～0
		Sanitation service	10	10～8	7～5	4～2	1～0
		Laundry service	10	10～8	7～5	4～2	1～0
		Haircut service	10	10～8	7～5	4～2	1～0
		Purchasing and mailing service	10	10～8	7～5	4～2	1～0

Table A. 3 （*continued*）

Evaluation item	Total score	Evaluation content	Score of sub-item	Excellent	Good	General	Poor
Basic conditions	700	Communication service	10	10～8	7～5	4～2	1～0
		Cultural and recreational services	10	10～8	7～5	4～2	1～0
		Psychological counseling/emotional support services	20	20～15	14～9	8～4	3～0
		Hospice care service	30	30～22	21～13	12～4	3～0
		Nutrition assessment service	10	10～8	7～5	4～2	1～0
		Nursing service	80	80～60	59～36	35～16	15～0
		Rehabilitation service	80	80～60	59～36	35～16	15～0
		Medical service	100	100～80	79～50	49～20	19～0
		Satisfaction on degree of combining medical and senior care services	30	30～22	21～13	12～4	3～0
		Office network	10	10～8	7～5	4～2	1～0
		Video network consultation service outside hospital	20	20～15	14～9	8～4	3～0
		Follow-up after discharge	10	10～8	7～5	4～2	1～0
		Service quality evaluation and improvement	10	10～8	7～5	4～2	1～0

A. 4 Basic conditions of assessment and grading criteria for grade-3 service institutions of combination of medical and enior health care are shownED in Table A. 4.

Table A. 4 Basic conditions of assessment and grading criteria for grade-3 service institutions of combination of medical and enior health care

Evaluation item	Total score	Evaluation content	Score of sub-item	Excellent	Good	General	Poor
Basic conditions	900	Scale of medical and nursing institutions	30	30～22	21～13	12～4	3～0
		Self-managed medical institution	30	30～22	21～13	12～4	3～0
		Affiliated hospital	20	20～15	14～9	8～4	3～0
		Nurse/patient ratio	30	30～22	21～13	12～4	3～0
		Proportion of nursing staff with professional titles in senior care	30	30～22	21～13	12～4	3～0
		Institutional occupancy rate	30	30～22	21～13	12～4	3～0
		In-and-out patient service	10	10～8	7～5	4～2	1～0
		Life assistance service	100	100～80	79～50	49～20	19～0

Table A.4（*continued*）

Evaluation item	Total score	Evaluation content	Score of sub-item	Excellent	Good	General	Poor
Basic conditions	900	Annual physical examination service for the elderly	10	10~8	7~5	4~2	1~0
		Dietary service	10	10~8	7~5	4~2	1~0
		Sanitation service	10	10~8	7~5	4~2	1~0
		Laundry service	10	10~8	7~5	4~2	1~0
		Haircut service	10	10~8	7~5	4~2	1~0
		Purchasing and mailing service	10	10~8	7~5	4~2	1~0
		Communication service	10	10~8	7~5	4~2	1~0
		Cultural and recreational services	10	10~8	7~5	4~2	1~0
		Physical fitness service	10	10~8	7~5	4~2	1~0
		Tourism service	10	10~8	7~5	4~2	1~0
		Psychological counseling/emotional support services	20	20~15	14~9	8~4	3~0
		Hospice care service	30	30~22	21~13	12~4	3~0
		Soothing medical services	30	30~22	21~13	12~4	3~0
		Nutrition assessment service	10	10~8	7~5	4~2	1~0
		Nursing service	80	80~60	59~36	35~16	15~0
		Rehabilitation service	80	80~60	59~36	35~16	15~0
		Rehabilitation and endowment traditional Chinese medicine	80	80~60	59~36	35~16	15~0
		Medical service	100	100~80	79~50	49~20	19~0
		Satisfaction on degree of combining medical and senior care services	30	30~22	21~13	12~4	3~0
		Office network	10	10~8	7~5	4~2	1~0
		Video network for out-of-hospital consultation service	20	20~15	14~9	8~4	3~0
		Follow-up after discharge	10	10~8	7~5	4~2	1~0
		Social worker service	10	10~8	7~5	4~2	1~0
		Evaluation and improvement of service quality	10	10~8	7~5	4~2	1~0

A.5 Basic conditions of assessment and grading criteria for grade-4 service institutions of combination of medical and enior health care are showned in Table A.5.

Table A. 5 Basic conditions of assessment and grading criteria for grade-4
service institutions of combination of medical and enior health care

Evaluation item	Total score	Evaluation content	Score of sub-item	Excellent	Good	General	Poor
Basic conditions	1 000	Scale of medical and nursing institutions	40	40~30	29~18	17~8	7~0
		Self-built medical institution	40	40~30	29~18	17~8	7~0
		Affiliated hospital	20	20~15	14~9	8~4	3~0
		Nurse/patient ratio	40	40~30	29~18	17~8	7~0
		Proportion of nursing staff with professional titles in senior care	40	40~30	29~18	17~8	7~0
		Institutional occupancy rate	40	40~30	29~18	17~8	7~0
		In-and-out patient service	10	10~8	7~5	4~2	1~0
		Life assistance service	100	100~80	79~50	49~20	19~0
		Annual physical examination service for the elderly	10	10~8	7~5	4~2	1~0
		Dietary service	10	10~8	7~5	4~2	1~0
		Sanitation service	10	10~8	7~5	4~2	1~0
		Laundry service	10	10~8	7~5	4~2	1~0
		Haircut service	10	10~8	7~5	4~2	1~0
		Purchasing and mailing service	10	10~8	7~5	4~2	1~0
		Communication service	10	10~8	7~5	4~2	1~0
		Cultural and recreational services	10	10~8	7~5	4~2	1~0
		University for the elderly	10	10~8	7~5	4~2	1~0
		Physical fitness service	10	10~8	7~5	4~2	1~0
		Tourism service	10	10~8	7~5	4~2	1~0
		Psychological counseling/emotional support services	20	20~15	14~9	8~4	3~0
		Hospice care service	30	30~22	21~13	12~4	3~0
		Soothing medical services	30	30~22	21~13	12~4	3~0
		Nutrition assessment service	10	10~8	7~5	4~2	1~0
		Nursing service	80	80~60	59~36	35~16	15~0
		Rehabilitation service	80	80~60	59~36	35~16	15~0
		Rehabilitation and endowment of traditional Chinese medicine	80	80~60	59~36	35~16	15~0
		Medical service	100	100~80	79~50	49~20	19~0
		Contracted domestic service	30	30~22	21~13	12~4	3~0

Table A. 5 (*continued*)

Evaluation item	Total score	Evaluation content	Score of sub-item	Excellent	Good	General	Poor
Basic conditions	1 000	Satisfaction on degree of combining medical and senior care services	30	30～22	21～13	12～4	3～0
		Office network service	10	10～8	7～5	4～2	1～0
		Network for medical consultations from reputable hospitals	30	30～22	21～13	12～4	3～0
		Follow-up after discharge	10	10～8	7～5	4～2	1～0
		Social worker service	10	10～8	7～5	4～2	1～0
		Evaluation and improvement of Service quality	10	10～8	7～5	4～2	1～0

A. 6 Basic conditions of assessment and grading criteria for grade 5 service institutions of combination of medical and enior health care are showned in Table A. 6.

Table A. 6 Basic conditions of assessment contents and grading criteria for grade 5 service institutions of combination of medical and enior health care

Evaluation item	Total score	Evaluation content	Score of sub-item	Excellent	Good	General	Poor
Basic conditions	1 100	Scale of medical and nursing institutions	50	50～40	39～25	24～10	9～0
		Self-built medical institution	50	50～40	39～25	24～10	9～0
		Affiliated hospital	30	30～22	21～13	12～4	3～0
		Nurse/patient ratio	50	50～40	39～25	24～10	9～0
		Proportion of nursing staff with professional titles in senior care	50	50～40	39～25	24～10	9～0
		Institutional occupancy rate	50	50～40	39～25	24～10	9～0
		In-and-out patient service	10	10～8	7～5	4～2	1～0
		Life assistance service	100	100～80	79～50	49～20	19～0
		Annual physical examination service for the elderly	20	20～15	14～9	8～4	3～0
		Dietary service	10	10～8	7～5	4～2	1～0
		Sanitation service	10	10～8	7～5	4～2	1～0
		Laundry service	10	10～8	7～5	4～2	1～0
		Haircut service	10	10～8	7～5	4～2	1～0
		Shopping and purchasing agent services	10	10～8	7～5	4～2	1～0
		Communication，post and telecommunications，postal services	10	10～8	7～5	4～2	1～0

Table A.6 (*continued*)

Evaluation item	Total score	Evaluation content	Score of sub-item	Excellent	Good	General	Poor
Basic conditions	1 100	Cultural and recreational services	10	10~8	7~5	4~2	1~0
		University for the elderly	10	10~8	7~5	4~2	1~0
		Physical fitness service	10	10~8	7~5	4~2	1~0
		Tourism, social services	10	10~8	7~5	4~2	1~0
		Landscaping and gardening service	10	10~8	7~5	4~2	1~0
		Psychological counseling/emotional support services	30	30~22	21~13	12~4	3~0
		Hospice care service	30	30~22	21~13	12~4	3~0
		Soothing medical services	30	30~22	21~13	12~4	3~0
		Nutritional assessment and guidance on dietary	20	20~15	14~9	8~4	3~0
		Nursing service	80	80~60	59~36	35~16	15~0
		Rehabilitation service	80	80~60	59~36	35~16	15~0
		Rehabilitation and endowment of traditional Chinese medicine	70	70~50	49~30	29~13	12~0
		Medical service	100	100~80	79~50	49~20	19~0
		Contracted domestic service	30	30~22	21~13	12~4	3~0
		Satisfaction on degree of combining medical and senior care services	30	30~22	21~13	12~4	3~0
		Office network service	10	10~8	7~5	4~2	1~0
		Network for medical consultations from reputable hospitals	30	30~22	21~13	12~4	3~0
		Follow-up after discharge	10	10~8	7~5	4~2	1~0
		Social worker service	10	10~8	7~5	4~2	1~0
		Evaluation and improvement of service quality	20	20~15	14~9	8~4	3~0

Bibliography

［1］ A3ZDYY-NY-20070924055，Classification and management standards of comphrehensive Hospitals（trial），National Ministry of Health

［2］ Basic standards for nursing homes（2011），National Ministry of Health

［3］ Code of conduct for employees in medical institutions（2012），National Ministry of Health

［4］ Basic Standards of infirmariy in ederly care institutions（trial）（2014），National Health and Family Planning Commission

［5］ Basic Standards of nursing stations in elderly care institutions（trial）（2014），National Health and Family Planning Commission

［6］ National code of basic public health services（3rd Edition）（2017），National Health and Family Planning Commission

［7］ T/CGSS 003—2018　Specification for age-friendly service

ICS 03.080
A 20

团　体　标　准

T/CGSS 007—2019

社区适老营养师规范

Specifications of community dietitians for the elderly

2019-10-14 发布

2019-10-14 实施

中国老年医学学会　发　布

前　言

本标准按照 GB/T 1.1—2009 给出的规则起草。

本标准由中国老年医学学会营养与食品安全分会、中国老年医学学会科技成果转化工作委员会、四川大学华西临床医学院/华西医院和四川华西健康教育咨询中心提出。

本标准由中国老年医学学会归口。

本标准起草单位：中国老年医学学会营养与食品安全分会、中国老年医学学会科技成果转化工作委员会、北京华仁适老安养咨询服务有限公司、四川大学华西临床医学院/华西医院、四川华西健康教育咨询中心、国家老年疾病临床医学研究中心（解放军总医院）、北京协和医院、解放军总医院、华中科技大学同济医学院附属同济医院、陆军军医大学大坪医院、海军军医大学、中国人民解放军联勤保障部队第903 医院、广西医科大学第一附属医院。

本标准主要起草人：胡雯、程志、于康、姚颖、郑延松、许红霞、缪明永、张勇胜、尤祥妹、裴耀东、吴砚荣、胡庆祥、孙静、刘春源、丁群芳、饶志勇、柳园、景小凡、李晶晶、程懿、王艳、于凤梅、石磊、蒲芳芳、薛宇、李雪梅、母东煜、袁红、马向华、刘英华、朱翠凤、施万英、周莉、李莉、江华、顾中一、陈永春、杨大刚、胡怀东、孙萍、翁敏、蒋志雄、张晓伟、洪东旭、张胜康、洪晶安、牟波、谭桂军、韩苏婷、孙明晓、邵春海、叶文锋、张明、张如富、孙丽娟、杨敏、毛金媛、王莹、吴琦、林根、陈水超、田文。

社区适老营养师规范

1 范围

本标准规定了社区适老营养师的分级、基本要求、服务要求、技能要求、培训及考核。

本标准适用于社区适老营养师的培训、考核与等级评定。

2 规范性引用文件

下列文件对于本文件的应用是必不可少的。凡是注日期的引用文件,仅注日期的版本适用于本文件。凡是不注日期的引用文件,其最新版本(包括所有的修改单)适用于本文件。

GB/T 20647.1—2006　社区服务指南　第1部分:总则

T/CGSS 004　适老营养配方食品通则

3 术语和定义

T/CGSS 004 界定的以及下列术语和定义适用于本文件。

3.1

营养师　dietitian

基于全人群、全生命周期的营养需要,科学运用膳食营养知识,提供全面营养管理的专业人员。

3.2

适老营养师　dietitians for the elderly

经过规范化培训并取得资质,为老年人实施营养教育、膳食营养实践和服务等全面营养管理的营养师。

3.3

社区　community

居住在一定地域内的人们所组成的各种社会关系的生活共同体。

[GB/T 20647.1—2006,定义3.1]

3.4

社区适老营养师　community dietitians for the elderly

为居住在一定地域内的人们所组成的各种社会关系的生活共同体、居家和医疗养老相关机构中老年人提供专业服务的适老营养师。

3.5

医院-家庭营养管理模式　hospital to home nutrition management mode;H2H

由医疗机构就职的营养师等医院医务人员联合社区相关工作人员及患者家属,把营养治疗从医院延续到院外,将单一治疗方式丰富为多形式治疗方案的管理模式。

4 社区适老营养师分级

社区适老营养师依据专业知识及技能分为三级,分别为初级、中级、高级。

5 基本要求

5.1 应具有中专/高中及以上学历,18周岁以上,具有完全民事行为能力。

5.2 应体检合格,持有二级及以上医疗机构出具的本人近3个月内的健康体检证明,无精神病史,无传染性疾病,具有正常的视觉、味觉和嗅觉能力,无影响执行社区适老营养师服务要求的疾病。

5.3 应遵守国家法律法规,熟悉《中华人民共和国老年人权益保障法》《中华人民共和国食品安全法》,具备为老年人提供专业服务的营养知识和技能。

6 服务要求

6.1 应提供营养健康教育服务。

6.2 应提供合理膳食指导服务,制定膳食配餐方案并监督实施。

6.3 应提供营养风险筛查服务,发现高风险人群并提供就诊建议。

6.4 在医疗机构的营养师指导下,应为出院康复期老年人提供膳食营养管理服务。

7 技能要求

7.1 概述

本标准对初、中、高各级的社区适老营养师的技能要求依次递进,高级别涵盖低级别。

7.2 初级社区适老营养师

7.2.1 符合a)或b)之一:

　　a) 应具有中专/高中及以上学历证书,经过初级社区适老营养师培训并考核合格者;

　　b) 应具有营养学/老年服务与管理/护理学/预防医学/临床医学等相关专业中专及以上学历,且实际从事社区适老营养工作满1年,经过初级社区适老营养师考核合格者。

7.2.2 掌握并具备基本的社区适老营养理论和实践操作技能:

　　a) 应掌握营养学基本知识和适老营养的基本原则,能够指导老年人日常膳食安排。

　　b) 应掌握肠内营养管的照护和管理相关技能,能够独立完成管饲。

　　c) 在专业人员的指导下,应能够协助实施以下工作:

　　　　1) 营养风险筛查;

　　　　2) 应用适老营养配方食品;

　　　　3) H2H流程。

　　d) 应参加社区适老营养师等级培训与技能实践,不少于240个学时并考核合格,具备基本的社区适老营养理论和实践操作技能。

7.3 中级社区适老营养师

7.3.1 符合a)或b)之一:

　　a) 应取得初级社区适老营养师资格后从事社区适老营养工作满2年以上,经中级社区适老营养师培训并考核合格者;

　　b) 应具有营养学/老年服务与管理/护理学/预防医学/临床医学等相关专业大专及以上学历,且实际从事社区适老营养工作满1年,或取得营养指导员资格证(中国营养学会颁发),经过中级社区适老营养师考核合格者。

7.3.2 在 7.2.2 基础上增加以下要求：

a) 应掌握营养风险筛查的技能，能够熟练运用营养风险筛查量表，独立完成筛查工作；

b) 应掌握适老营养配方食品的应用原则，能够应用适老营养配方食品；

c) 应掌握老年人常见疾病的膳食营养原则，能够独立对患病老年人进行个体化营养教育和指导；

d) 应熟悉 H2H 的流程，能够建立和管理老年人家庭营养档案，收集和录入基本信息；

e) 应参加社区适老营养师等级培训与技能实践，不少于 180 个学时并考核合格，具备较高的社区适老营养理论和实践操作技能。

7.4 高级社区适老营养师

7.4.1 符合 a)或 b)之一：

a) 应取得中级社区适老营养师资格后从事社区适老营养工作满 2 年，经高级社区适老营养师培训并考核合格者；

b) 应具有营养学/老年服务与管理/护理学/预防医学/临床医学等相关专业本科及以上学历，且实际从事社区适老营养工作满 1 年，或取得注册营养师资格证（中国营养学会颁发），经过高级社区适老营养师考核合格者。

7.4.2 在 7.3.2 基础上增加以下要求：

a) 应熟悉营养评价流程，能够灵活应用常用营养评价量表；

b) 应掌握 H2H 的流程，能够独立对老年人进行定期营养随访和监测；

c) 应熟悉肠内/肠外营养治疗原则，能够为适用人群/慎用人群提供建议；

d) 应熟悉转诊流程，能够对存在营养问题的老年人提供就医建议；

e) 应参加社区适老营养师等级培训与技能实践，不少于 120 个学时并考核合格，具备全面的社区适老营养理论和实践操作技能。

8 培训及考核

8.1 应参加由中国老年医学学会组织的社区适老营养师等级培训项目，根据不同等级完成规定学时。

8.2 由中国老年医学学会组织"社区适老营养师"考核，经考核合格的人员，颁发中国老年医学学会"社区适老营养师"等级证书。

8.3 各级社区适老营养师取得合格证书后，每年应参加社区适老营养师指定培训不少于 24 个学时。

8.4 社区适老营养师等级证书信息在中国老年医学学会指定网站发布。

8.5 获得社区适老营养师等级证书后，若有医疗、卫生、职业道德等违法违规行为，将被取消其所获证书资质并予以通报。

————————————

ICS 03.080
A 20

Social Organization Standard

T/CGSS 007—2019

Specification of community dietitians for the elderly

社区适老营养师规范

(English Translation)

Issue date：2019-10-14   **Implementation date**：2019-10-14

Issued by   Chinese Geriatrics Society

Foreword

This standard was drafted in accordance with the rules given in the GB/T 1. 1—2009.

This standard was proposed by Department of Nutrition and Food Safety of Chinese Geriatrics Society, Committee on Scientific Transformation and Technological Achievement of Chinese Geriatrics Society, West China School of Medicine of Sichuan University/West China Hospital and Sichuan West China Health Consulting center.

This standard was prepared by Chinese Geriatrics Society.

This standard was drafted by the Department of Nutrition and Food Safety of Chinese Geriatrics Society, Committee on Scientific Transformation and Technological Achievementof Chinese Geriatrics Society, West China School of Medicine of Sichuan University/West China Hospital, Sichuan West China Health Consulting center, National Clinical Research Center of Geriatrics Disease (Chinese PLA General Hospital), Peking Union Medical College Hospital, Chinese PLA General Hospital, Tongji Hospital of Tongji Medical College of Huazhong University of Science and Technology, Daping Hospital of Army Medical University; The Second Military Medical University, 903rd Hospital of PLA Joint Logistics Support Force and The First Affiliated Hospital of Guangxi Medical University.

The main drafters of this standard were WenHu, Zhi Cheng, Kang Yu, Ying Yao, Yansong Zheng, Hongxia Xu, Mingyong Miu, Yongsheng Zhang, Xiangmei You, Yaodong Qiu, Yanrong Wu, Qingxiang Hu, Jing Sun, Chunyuan Liu, Qunfang Ding, Zhiyong Yao, Yuan Liu, Xiaofan Jing, Jingjing Li, Yi Cheng, Yan Wang, Fengmei Yu, Lei Shi, Fangfang Pu, Yu Xue, Xuemei Li, Dongyu Mu, Hong Yuan, Xianghua Ma, Yinghua Liu, Cuifeng Zhu, Wanying Shi, Li Zhou, Li Li, Hua Jiang, Zhongyi Gu, Yongchun Chen, Dagang Yang, Huaidong Hu, Ping Sun, Min Weng, Zhixiong Jiang, Xiaowei Zhang, Dongxu Hong, Shengkang Zhang, Jingan Hong, Bo Mu, Guijun Tan, Suting Han, Mingxiao Sun, Chunhai Shao, Wenfeng Ye, Ming Zhang, Rufu Zhang, Lijuan Sun, Min Yang, Jinyuan Mao, Ying Wang, Qi Wu, Gen Lin, Shui chao Chen and Wen Tian.

Specification of community dietitians for the elderly

1　Scope

This standard specifies the classification, basic requirements, service requirements, skills requirements, training and assessment of community dieticians for the elderly. This standard is applicable to the training, assessment and grading of dieticians for the elderly.

2　Normative references

The following referenced documents are indispensable for the application of this document. For dated references, only the edition cited applies. For undated references, the latest edition of the referenced document (including any amendments) applies.

T/CGSS 004　General rules of nutrition formula food for the elderly.

3　Terms and definitions

For the purposes of this document, the terms and definitions given in T/CGSS 004 and the following apply.

3.1
dietitian

the professionals applying scientific dietary and nutrition knowledge to provide comprehensive management on diet to accommendate the nutritional needs of total population and human life cycle

3.2
dietitian for the elderly

the dietitians professionally trained and qualifed for the implementation of nutrition education, dietary nutrition practice, and comprehensive nutrition management for the elderly

3.3
community

a social network formed by people living in a certain area

[GB/T 20647. 1—2006,definition 3. 1]

3. 4
community dietitians for the elderly

the dietitians professionally trained and qualifed for the implementation of nutrition education,dietary nutrition practice and comprehensive nutrition management for the elderly who live in a certain area of social network or in a certain nursing and care service institution

3. 5
hospital to home nutrition management mode
H2H

a nutrition management plan conducted by medical staff such as hospital dietitians in joint effort with other community service providers or patient family members that connects nutrition treatments in hospital to in-home dietary services and provide the elderly the intergrated dietary guidance and more options for in-home services

4 Grade levels of community dietitians for the elderly

Based on professional knowledge and skills,community dietitians for the elderly can be graded as entry-level,intermediate-level and advanced-level.

5 Basic requirements

5. 1 At least a high school or equivalent secondary technical diploma required,above theage of 18, and shall have full civil legal capacity.

5. 2 Shall pass the physical examinations with a health certificate issued within 3 months by qualified medical institutions. Shall have no medical history of any mental illness,infectious disease,loss of vision,loss of sensations or diseases and disabilities affecting work performance of a community dietitian.

5. 3 Shall comply with national laws and regulations,master the knowledge of *Law of the People's Republic of China on the Protection of Rights and Interests of the Elderly*, *Food Safety Law of the People's Republic of China*,and shall have nutrition knowledge and relevant skills to provide professional services for the elderly.

6 Service requirements

6. 1 Shall provide nutrition and health education services.

6.2 Shall provide customized dietary guidance, design meal plans, and provide supervison on meal plan implementation.

6.3 Provide risk screening services to identify thehigh-risk elderly populations, and provide further medical and treatment suggestions.

6.4 With guidance from clinical dietitians, community dietitians shall provide extended nutrition management services for the elderly discharged from the hospital.

7　Skill requirements

7.1　Overview

This standard provides guidelines for entry-level, intermediate-level and advanced-level community dietitians. The required capability increases as the grade level increases.

7.2　Entry-level requirements

7.2.1　a) or b):

a)　At least have a high school or equivalent secondary technical diploma required, and havepassed the entry-level qualification exam for community dietitians.

b)　At least have a secondary technical diploma in fields of nutrition, elderly care service and management, nursing, preventive medicine or clinical medicine required, with at least one-year work experience of community elderly care service, and have passed the entry-level qualification exam for community dietitians.

7.2.2　Shall master basic knowledge of community nutrition and practical skills:

a)　Basic knowledge of nutrition and basic principles of nutrition for the elderly required, and capable of providing guidance on the elderly's daily diet.

b)　Relevant skills of care and management of enteral feeding tube uses, and capable of operating independently enteral tube feeding.

c)　Be able to assist in the operation of 1), 2) and 3) under the guidance of professionals:

1)　Nutrition risk screening,

2)　Utilize nutritional formula food for the elderly,

　　　3） H2H process.

d） Shall participate in no less than 240 hours of training for certain grade level and skill practice for community dietitians,and have passed the qualification exam. Master basic knowledge and practical skills of community dietitians.

7.3 Intermediate-level requirements

7.3.1 a）or b）:

a） Have certified for community dietitian practice,with 2 or more years of community dietitian experience,and have passed intermediate-level qualification exams.

b） At least have a bachelor or equivalent college degree in nutrition,elderly care service and management,nursing,preventive medicine or clinical medicine required,and with at least one-year work experience of community elderly care service or with certification of nutrition instructor by Chinese Nutrition Society,and have passed the intermediate-level qualification exam for community dietitians.

7.3.2 Shall meet the following requirements on the basis of 7.2.2:

a） Master nutrition risk screening skills,and be able to use nutrition risk screening scale and complete independently risk screening process.

b） Master application principles of nutritional formula food for the elderly,and be able toprovide nutritional formula food for the elderly.

c） Master general nutrition principles to provide customized diet for the elderly,and be able to provide independently customized guidance on diet for the elderly with illness.

d） Be familiar with H2H process,be able to establish and manage the archive system of family nutrition records of the elderly,and be able to collect and archive basic information.

e） Shall participate in no less than 180 hours of training for certain grade level and skill practice for community dieticians,and have passed the qualification exam. Master basic knowledge and practical skills required for higer level community dietitians.

7.4 Advanced-level requirements

7.4.1 a）or b）:

a） Have certified for intermediate-level community dietitian practice,with 2 or more years of community dietitian experience,and have passeded advanced-level qualification exams.

b) At least have a bachelor degree in nutrition,elderly care service and management,nursing,preventive medicine or clinical medicine required,and with at least one-year work experience of community elderly care service or with certification of nutrition instructor by Chinese Nutrition Society,and havepassed the advanced-level qualification exam for community dietitians.

7.4.2 Shall meetthe following requirements on the basis of 7.3.2:

a) Be familiar with nutrition evaluation process,and beable to apply commonly used nutrition evaluation scale.

b) Master H2H process and be able to conductindependently nutrition follow-up and monitoring for the elderly on a regular basis.

c) Be familiar with the use principles of enteral/parenteral nutrition feeding,and capable of providing suggestions for the elderly with certain indications and precautions.

d) Be familiar with referral process and be able to provide medical advice to the elderly with nutritional concerns.

e) Shall participate in no less than 120 hours of training for certain grade level and skill practice for community dieticians,and havepassed the qualification exam. Master basic knowledge and practical skills required for higer level community dietitians.

8 Training and assessment

8.1 Community dietitians for the elderlyshall attend the training programs provided by Chinese geriatrics society. Based on the grade level,the required training hours vary.

8.2 The certificate of community dietitians for the elderlywill be issued by Chinese geriatrics society upon passing the qualification exams.

8.3 All grade level community dietitians for the elderlyshall continue to have at least 24 hours of training for community dietitians after obtaining the certification.

8.4 The information of certificate of community dietitians for the elderlywill be released on the official website ofChinese Geriatrics Society.

8.5 The certificateof community dietitiansfor the elderly will be suspended upon any misconduct in medical and healthcare practice or ethics of the certification holder.

———————————